Advance Praise for
DSM-5® Pocket Guide for Child and Adolescent Mental Health

"This book is a compendium, in 300 pages, of practical clinical wisdom regarding the assessment and treatment of psychiatric problems in children and adolescents. It is a highly useful translation and expansion of DSM-5 for the pediatric population, where familial, developmental, environmental, and contextual factors make the diagnostic process especially challenging. Drs. Hilt and Nussbaum's calm and exquisitely clear prose makes this volume a delight to read no matter what one's discipline or level of training."

> *Gregory K. Fritz, M.D., Professor and Director, Division of Child and Adolescent Psychiatry, and Vice Chair, Department of Psychiatry and Human Behavior, Warren Alpert Medical School of Brown University; Academic Director, E.P. Bradley Hospital; and Associate Chief and Director of Child Psychiatry, Rhode Island Hospital/Hasbro Children's Hospital*

"This book takes an intensely practical approach to initial diagnosis and management of behavioral health problems in children and youth, making it useful for any clinician who provides care to children in an outpatient setting. It has the same degree of empathy for the clinicians using it that we all hope to provide for the children and families we care for."

> *Christopher Stille, M.D., M.P.H., Professor and Section Head, General Academic Pediatrics, University of Colorado School of Medicine/Children's Hospital Colorado*

"Robert Hilt and Abraham Nussbaum have written an efficient and effective guide to the mental health interview and use of DSM-5 with children and adolescents. Together with the handy tables provided regarding treatments, this summary and explanation of the DSM-5 diagnostic criteria and detailed guide to the clinical interview will be useful to all clinicians working with youth, especially those in primary care. The authors emphasize that when evaluating a young patient, the practitioner must consider all aspects, not only of the patient, but also of the family, school, and community, and develop the relationship before launching into a symptom checklist."

Mina K. Dulcan, M.D., Head, Child and Adolescent Psychiatry, Ann & Robert H. Lurie Children's Hospital of Chicago, and Professor of Psychiatry and Behavioral Sciences and Pediatrics, Northwestern University Feinberg School of Medicine

"Hilt and Nussbaum's DSM-5 Pocket Guide is an outstanding, user -friendly, clinically meaningful interpretation of disorders relevant to those of us evaluating and treating children and adolescents. It provides not only youth-specific information on the disorders; it provides very useful ways of soliciting the information as well as guidelines for treatment planning and psychopharmacologic and psychosocial treatments. Think of the volume as cutting the huge plate of child and adolescent diagnosis, psychopathology, and treatment into bite-sized and easy to swallow pieces! Clinicians caring for the mental health of children shouldn't be without it!"

Gabrielle A. Carlson, M.D., Professor of Psychiatry and Pediatrics, Stony Brook University School of Medicine, Putnam Hall-South Campus

DSM-5®
POCKET GUIDE
FOR
CHILD AND ADOLESCENT MENTAL HEALTH

DSM-5®
POCKET GUIDE
FOR
CHILD AND
ADOLESCENT
MENTAL HEALTH

Robert J. Hilt, M.D., FAAP, FAACAP, FAPA

*Associate Professor, Department of Psychiatry,
University of Washington, and Director, Partnership
Access Line, Seattle Children's Hospital,
Seattle, Washington*

Abraham M. Nussbaum, M.D., FAPA

*Director, Denver Health Adult Inpatient Psychiatry,
and Assistant Professor, Department of Psychiatry,
University of Colorado School of Medicine,
Denver, Colorado*

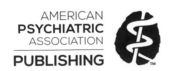

AMERICAN
PSYCHIATRIC
ASSOCIATION
PUBLISHING

If you wish to buy 50 or more copies of the same title, please go to www.appi.org/specialdiscounts for more information.

Copyright © 2016 American Psychiatric Association Publishing

ALL RIGHTS RESERVED

DSM and DSM-5 are registered trademarks of the American Psychiatric Association. Use of these terms is prohibited without permission of the American Psychiatric Association.

Manufactured in the United States of America on acid-free paper
21 20   7   6
First Edition

American Psychiatric Association Publishing
800 Maine Avenue SW, Suite 900
Washington, DC 20024
www.appi.org

Library of Congress Cataloging-in-Publication Data
Hilt, Robert J., 1969– , author.
  DSM-5 pocket guide for child and adolescent mental health / by Robert J. Hilt, Abraham M. Nussbaum.
    p. ; cm.
  Pocket guide for child and adolescent mental health
  Diagnostic and statistical manual of mental disorders-5 pocket guide for child and adolescent mental health
  Diagnostic and statistical manual of mental disorders-five pocket guide for child and adolescent mental health
  Includes bibliographical references and index.
  ISBN 978-1-58562-494-2 (pb : alk. paper)
  I. Nussbaum, Abraham M., 1975– , author. II. American Psychiatric Association, issuing body. III. Title. IV. Title: Pocket guide for child and adolescent mental health. V. Title: Diagnostic and statistical manual of mental disorders-5 pocket guide for child and adolescent mental health. VI. Title: Diagnostic and statistical manual of mental disorders-five pocket guide for child and adolescent mental health.
  [DNLM: 1. Diagnostic and statistical manual of mental disorders. 5th ed. 2. Mental Disorders—diagnosis—Handbooks. 3. Mental Disorders—therapy—Handbooks. 4. Adolescent. 5. Child. 6. Interview, Psychological—methods—Handbooks. WS 39]
  RJ503
  616.8900835—dc23   2015031532

British Library Cataloguing in Publication Data
A CIP record is available from the British Library.

Contents

Preface vii

SECTION I
DIAGNOSING AND TREATING CHILDREN AND ADOLESCENTS

1 Introduction 3

2 Addressing Behavioral and Mental
Problems in Community Settings. 9

3 Common Clinical Concerns 21

4 The 15-Minute
Pediatric Diagnostic Interview 59

5 The 30-Minute
Pediatric Diagnostic Interview 71

SECTION II
USING DSM-5 WITH CHILDREN AND ADOLESCENTS

6 DSM-5 Pediatric
Diagnostic Interview 83

7 A Brief Version of DSM-5 175

SECTION III

ADDITIONAL TOOLS
AND CLINICAL GUIDANCE

8 A Stepwise Approach
to Differential Diagnosis. 189

9 The Mental Status Examination:
A Psychiatric Glossary 195

10 Selected DSM-5
Assessment Measures 199

11 Rating Scales and
Alternative Diagnostic Systems 227

12 Developmental Milestones 241

13 Mental Health Treatment Planning 249

14 Psychosocial Interventions. 257

15 Psychotherapeutic Interventions 267

16 Psychopharmacological Interventions . . . 275

17 Ideas for Practice,
Education, and Research 301

References. 305

Index 315

Preface

The release of DSM-5 occasioned a renewed interest in how to evaluate a person in mental distress for the presence of a mental disorder (e.g., American Psychiatric Association 2015; Lieberman 2015; Phillips et al. 2012a, 2012b, 2012c). Such an evaluation can seem impossible. After all, when you are determining whether a person is experiencing a mental disorder, you consider many aspects of a person, including his or her culture, ethnicity, faith, family history, gender, medical history, sexual orientation, and temperament. When making those determinations in children and adolescents, your evaluation is often even more complex. You must know both a person's age and his or her developmental age. You must know both a person's temperament and the temperament of his or her parents. You must know the health of a person and the health of his or her family.

By design, DSM-5 is a manual for the diagnosis of mental illness in a particular person, so using it in children and adolescents, whose health is inevitably bound up in the communities and families in which they are situated, requires an act of translation. This manual is, itself, a pragmatic translation of DSM-5. This book is not a replacement for DSM-5 itself or the many pediatric psychiatric interview textbooks (e.g., Cepeda 2010; Mash and Barkley 2007) but a way to use the DSM-5 criteria as part of a diagnostic interview to guide treatment planning.

Every day we interview patients with students, trainees, and fellow practitioners, so we wrote the book for interviewers at all levels of experience. The first section of the book introduces the diagnostic interview, its goals, and how to structure an interview according to how much time you have with a person. The second section operationalizes the DSM-5 diagnostic criteria for clinical practice. The third section includes additional information, tables, and tools. Taken as a whole, this book helps you accurately diagnose mental disorders in a child or an adolescent while establishing a therapeutic alliance, which remains the goal of any psychiatric encounter.

Before we begin, a few words about the language we use in this book. When possible, we use neutral gender for the person and the interviewer, but when doing so is grammatically awkward, we alternate between the universal feminine in odd-numbered chapters and the universal masculine in the even-numbered chapters.

Wherever possible, we emphasize the agency, the ability of a child or an adolescent to act in the world. To signal this emphasis, we use the word *person* to describe the object of mental health evaluation. We acknowledge that a robust debate exists about whether the object of medical care is best construed as an ill patient under the care of a health professional or as an autonomous consumer of that professional's services (cf. Emanuel and Emanuel 1992), but because personhood precedes illness or consumption, we prefer *person*. However, when we write about a person who has entered psychiatric treatment, we use the term *patient* because it acknowledges both the vulnerability of the person in treatment and the responsibilities assumed by professionals when they care for patients (cf. Radden and Sadler 2010). We use the term *patient* not to endorse medical paternalism but to emphasize that the particular and protected relationships that develop in clinical encounters are better described as therapeutic relationships rather than as therapeutic contracts.

Because children and adolescents often depend on a variety of adults—parents, extended family members, adult friends, teachers, faith leaders, coaches, and more—for their needs, we use the term *caregiver* to describe an adult who cares for a child or an adolescent outside of medical relationships.

Finally, we are both physicians, but children and adolescents receive care within medical relationships from persons trained in a variety of helping professions. To acknowledge this variety, we use the term *practitioner* to describe a medical professional who cares for children and adolescents. Although *provider* is the more common euphemism, we prefer *practitioner* because it emphasizes the ways a professional who meets children and adolescents as patients is constantly practicing and refining his or her craft.

Acknowledgments

We thank the teachers and students with whom we learned (and still learn) how to care for children and adolescents in mental distress, our respective academic and clinical homes for encouraging this work, and our own families for tolerating our efforts.

The authors have no competing interests or conflicts to declare.

SECTION I

Diagnosing and Treating Children and Adolescents

Chapter 1

Introduction

In the midst of an overbooked afternoon, you are asked to perform a mental health assessment of Sophie, a 14-year-old girl you have never met. You gather some materials, enter her examination room, and find a poorly groomed girl with her arms crossed over her chest, staring up at the ceiling rather than looking at you. She says to no one in particular, "There is nothing wrong, and I don't need to be here." Her mother then speaks for her, describing school struggles, arguments at home, losing friends, and saying "strange" things that include threats to hurt herself and talking to no one in particular whenever she is alone. She has a history of maltreatment by her mother's previous boyfriend, and in subsequent years she has had "mood swings." Sophie is picking at the scabs overlaying the linear lacerations on her left forearm.

That sinking feeling you just experienced—the time-stressed challenge of assessing mental health concerns in a pediatric population—is something we have experienced too. We want this book to help, to be the guide you take with you on these kinds of encounters.

What Is in This Book?

Like *The Pocket Guide to the DSM-5™ Diagnostic Exam*, this book emphasizes a person-centered approach to diagnosis along with practical tools and interview prompts to try with children and with their parents.

Because young people are more likely to receive an initial mental health diagnosis and medication management in a primary care setting than in a specialty care setting, we pay particular attention throughout this guide to what would be practical to perform in a primary care setting. Therefore, we describe things such as

- How to diagnostically investigate common complaints (Chapter 3)
- How to perform either 15-minute (Chapter 4) or 30-minute (Chapter 5) versions of a diagnostic interview
- Abbreviated DSM-5 (American Psychiatric Association 2013) diagnostic descriptions and criteria (Table 4–1 and Chapter 7)
- Rating scales and suggested uses (Chapters 10 and 11)
- Developmental milestones and red flags for referral (Chapters 3 and 12)
- Psychosocial (Chapter 14) and psychotherapeutic (Chapter 15) intervention basics
- Psychopharmacological intervention basics (Chapter 16)

We expect that different parts of this book will be used in different ways. Some sections of this book will be more helpful when read in their entirety because they describe strategies to approach different aspects of caring for young people. Other sections may be used as in-the-moment references, such as interview questions to try when investigating a specific DSM-5 diagnosis or a table that lists key age-specific developmental milestones.

The following points highlight how this book differs from *The Pocket Guide to the DSM-5™ Diagnostic Exam*.

- ICD-10 codes for diagnoses are included.
- Diagnoses not commonly made in childhood or adolescence are not included. All content is focused specifically on children and adolescents.
- Discussion of the development of DSM-5 is reduced because it is no longer novel.
- The practical aspects of the text are increased by shortening chapters and adding tables.
- Assessment tools specifically for children and adolescents are introduced.
- Initial treatment strategies—psychosocial, psychotherapeutic, and psychopharmacological—for diagnosed disorders are added.

We certainly did not start out knowing how to interview young people and diagnose their mental and behavioral health problems. We remember struggling through encounters, wondering how to organize the disparate symptoms and concerns. Through our struggles, we eventually arrived at a variety of ways to simplify the diagnostic and treatment process and have learned how to organize our approach even in time-constrained circumstances.

As coauthors, we have served in different postresidency clinical roles that include being a rural pediatrician, a pediatric hospitalist, a pediatric emergency physician, a child psychiatrist, a child psychiatric consultant to both tertiary care and rural pediatricians, and an adult inpatient psychiatrist. We have provided both psychotherapy and medication treatments for young people and have been required to adapt what we do for the shifting needs and structures of various care settings. In the course of this work, we have often been humbled by the challenges young people face and the challenges they present to a person who dares to provide them with mental health assistance. After all, few children and adolescents arrive on our doorsteps with neatly described symptoms that perfectly map onto a single DSM-5 disorder. We have both made many mistakes and grown from those experiences.

This book is an experience-based guide to child mental health diagnosis and treatment, intended to provide a variety of practical approaches, tips, and skills to supplement the diagnostic content of DSM-5. We cannot offer any rigid rules to follow when diagnosing or treating mental health disorders in young people because good care for young people cannot be reduced to a checklist. However, we make it easier for everyone to provide excellent care. Whatever your specialty, your practice setting, and your experience level, we can assist you as you journey with children and adolescents in pursuit of mental health.

Therapeutic Alliance: The Place to Start

Working with young people can be very different from working with adults. Young people are often reluctant participants, often with developmentally limited communication skills, who have been presented for care that they did not seek on their own. In addition, the process of diagnosing disorders in a child typically involves gathering information from multiple informants and remembering an age- and developmentally adjusted–diagnostic differential. Particularly when clinicians are working in primary care or other settings that artificially limit evaluation times, that sense of a ticking clock increases the challenges in order to efficiently reach a diagnosis and treatment plan for a young person.

The first step to successful diagnosis and treatment is to support the collaborative treatment relationship, what we hereinafter call the *therapeutic alliance*. Creating a therapeutic alliance with the caregiver at an appointment is comparatively simple when compared with building an alliance directly with a young person.

The 14-year-old girl in the vignette at the beginning of this chapter, Sophie, illustrates the problem with building an alliance. Sophie communicated that she disagreed with her mother's assessment of the situation and was disinterested in your services. If you were to open DSM-5 and immediately begin asking Sophie a series of diagnostic questions, it would likely only increase her resistance. You must first engage Sophie to obtain reliable responses.

If we were in the examination room with you, we would hear out the concerns of Sophie's mother, which also serves to solidify the parental therapeutic alliance; we would thank her for the guidance; and we would tell her that after hearing the concerns of caregivers, we speak with all of our adolescent patients alone. We would describe the rules for that discussion—namely, that the conversation is confidential except for safety concerns—and then invite Sophie to sit alone with us. We do so because with adolescents in particular, you develop a better alliance and obtain more honest answers when you interview them without a parent or caregiver present (cf. Ford et al. 1997; Gold and Seningen 2009). However, this guidance must be adapted to each situation; a separation should not be forced on an adolescent who does not want her or his caregivers to leave the room. Younger children, or those adolescents who appear to be developmentally immature, are usually interviewed more successfully with caregivers present and reassuring them.

All young people will have a better therapeutic alliance if they feel noticed, heard, and appreciated, which can be called *empathic engagement*. Even for practitioners in a time-pressured situation, be reassured that holding back a recitation of targeted diagnostic questions in order to really notice the patient and build a little engagement does not take long. In our experience, creating that engaged therapeutic alliance up front with a reluctant interviewee saves time overall through enhanced cooperation with the diagnostic process.

Starting with a genuine reflecting statement that follows someone's lead can initiate engagement with an adolescent, such as saying to Sophie, *"You said that you feel fine and that there is nothing wrong. I would like to hear more about what is going well for you right now...."* You could also start the conversation by asking about something that is important to the patient but relatively situation neutral, such as, *"Your mom said that you go to _____ school; what is that school like?"* School, friends, family, and favorite activities can all be appropriate and relatively low-stress conversation starters.

For young persons who seem really reluctant to even start talking, you may find that the conversation flows better after describing something you saw. This shows that you have been paying attention to them. For instance, *"It looked as if it was really hard to just sit there and do nothing while your mom was talking. Am I right about that?"* If there is a chance to comment on something you saw that relates to the diagnostic theme, you could also take that opportunity, saying, for example, *"I saw you shake your head when your mom described what happened yesterday. Did she say something that wasn't true for you?"*

With a very young child, a conversation starter could be a simple observation, such as commenting about what she is wearing or brought with her, such as, *"I see you have flowers on your shoes; did you pick those out yourself?"* You can also comment on something the young person is currently doing, such as how she is playing with a toy or drawing a picture, to start a conversation.

A more subtle strategy to build the treatment alliance with a young person is shaping how you speak in a way that shows that you will be a responsive, problem-solving partner rather than an authority who will judge her. Metaphorically, this is about getting you and your young patient to sit side by side and to talk about a problem together. That way, the young person can talk about a problem that does not involve who she is as a person. For instance, Sophie may feel less defensive if you conversationally refer to her "mood" having led her to cut herself rather than "you cut yourself."

A bit of humor can help to get young people talking. If humor does not come easily to you, be aware that showing some humility about yourself can be disarming and get your patient to chuckle a little. Both of us have children of our own who daily remind us that we have not been "cool" for a long time (if we ever were), and we find that openly acknowledging our status as uncool adults can humanize us and put a young person at ease. For instance, *"What is that band's name on your shirt? ... I have not heard about them before, but that probably means they are cool because I am a bit of a square."*

Building a therapeutic alliance with a young person should lead to learning that young patient's own true chief complaint. For Sophie, it could be "My mom is driving me crazy," "My boyfriend is abusive," "I hear voices," or any of a number of complaints. This creates a context from which your subsequent and more detailed diagnostic inquiries will logically follow. Following conversational opportunities can go like this: *"So, during those times when your mom is driving you crazy, do you ever have thoughts about hurting yourself?"* Child and parent chief complaints do not have to align; we have performed many successful treatments from start to finish with young people whose chief complaints never fully aligned with what their parents thought the problem was.

Once you have the young person engaged and talking with you, the diagnostic and treatment process as described throughout the rest of this book should follow along more easily. Once a reasonable therapeutic alliance has been started, it is our experience that asking your patient questions about what she sees as the challenges in her life will be more honestly answered.

In summary, we suggest the following techniques to initiate a therapeutic alliance with a child and set up a useful diagnostic interview:

- When developmentally appropriate, offer to talk with the patient without a caregiver present.
- Start the conversation with an observation or a subject important to the patient.
- Briefly convey that you have noticed, heard, and appreciated the patient's perspective.
- Show that you are the child's treatment partner rather than an adult-engaged adjudicator.
- Use a little humor to break the ice, such as confessing your "uncoolness."
- Ask about the patient's main concerns or frustrations.
- Try shaping your initial diagnostic questions to reference the child's own chief complaint.

Chapter 2

Addressing Behavioral and Mental Problems in Community Settings

Children infrequently receive timely care for mental and behavioral health problems: the average time from the start of child mental health symptoms until a young person enters mental health treatment is 8–10 years (Kessler et al. 2005). In many systems of care, only about one in five children with a diagnosable mental health disorder will receive treatment during childhood (U.S. Public Health Service Office of the Surgeon General 1999). For those children identified in primary care to be in need of a behavioral health intervention, a little more than half of those referred to a specialist will attend even a single treatment appointment (Rushton et al. 2002).

The reasons for this underuse of specific mental health treatments during childhood are numerous. Barriers include stigma, poor problem recognition, limited family or practitioner understanding of treatments, insurance coverage barriers, complicated referral processes, and limited availability of mental health specialists.

There are far more community issues to address than any of us as individual practitioners could change all at once. Thankfully, opportunities are now increasing for practitioners to participate in meaningful improvements in community behavioral health systems. Through payer supports and system redesigns, primary care practices may be able to develop collaborative or integrated care partnerships with mental health specialists. Doing so brings specialist support directly into sites where people are already receiving medical services. Research has determined that such arrangements can be clinically more effective and even save money for the overall care system, which has captured the attention of health systems and payers.

Regardless of the specific system of care available in your community, we would like to point out certain general clinical steps that appear along the path of addressing child behavioral health problems in community settings. If you are a primary care practitioner or a health system representative working to improve community behavioral health, identifying opportunities to improve any of the following areas is likely to improve the health of children:

- Recognition of mental distress
- Screening for mental distress
- Diagnosis of a particular mental disorder
- Education about mental health treatment
- Teaching patients and caregivers self-help strategies
- Initiation of counseling and therapy
- Appropriate prescription of medications

Recognition of Mental Distress

Before a child can receive services, he or she first must be *recognized* as needing some form of assistance. We point this out because caregivers have wide variations in their view of what requires professional help. The same set of disruptive behaviors may lead one caregiver to write it off as "Oh, he's just being a boy" but lead another caregiver to demand immediately to see a professional. Families may actively resist acknowledging or may simply fail to recognize when the child has a problem that treatment could help. Therefore, a key initial step in the process is for family members, friends, school representatives, and primary care practitioners to help parents recognize what can and cannot be helped through mental health treatment and overcome stigma barriers when necessary. Education about general signs of trouble to watch for—such as decreasing school performance or losing the ability to have fun—can aid with problem recognition.

Screening for Mental Distress

Proactively looking for mental health problems through direct questioning or evaluating symptoms with a behavioral health rating scale is worthwhile, but only if practitioners are available to interpret that information and recommend appropriate actions. Rating scales are very useful for their ease of administration and ability to identify unrecognized problems, to obtain clinical data from multiple informants, and to provide assessments of symptom severity to follow.

Rating scales are also inherently imperfect; they should never be the sole basis for making a diagnosis. This is because questions might be misinterpreted, might be answered untruthfully, or might simply have been the wrong questions to ask. For instance, an adolescent with recent-onset inattention problems may have a depressive disorder or an anxiety disorder missed if the only diagnostic assessment was an attention-deficit/hyperactivity (ADHD) disorder symptom rating scale. An adolescent who denies having depressive symptoms on a rating scale but is engaging in recurrent self-harm should still receive specialized care. Thus, the most valuable steps in a rating scale screening process are practitioners helping to select the correct scales, interpreting the results in the context of a person's personal situation, and taking a helpful action for any positive screening results.

Diagnosis of a Particular Mental Disorder

Making a mental health diagnosis and developing a treatment plan can be challenging for a mental health care practitioner who has up to an hour to complete his or her assessment. For those who are less experienced or have only 15 minutes to assess a person, the task quickly becomes overwhelming. Within a strictly limited and very short time frame, all that we would reasonably ask of a clinician is to identify the child's leading problem and its probable rather than definitive origin.

A well-supported DSM-5 (American Psychiatric Association 2013) diagnosis subsequently requires three things: 1) that a child's clinical presentation fulfills the specific symptom-based diagnostic criteria, 2) that those symptoms are not caused by other diagnoses or stressors, and 3) that those symptoms are impairing a child's functioning. Because challenges occur at each step, we recommend breaking up the process into several steps. In an initial brief assessment with incomplete information, we recommend that clinicians consider using less specific diagnoses, such as disruptive behavior disorder, unspecified, or depressive disorder, unspecified.

The diagnosis then can be clarified over time through gathering more information at subsequent appointments. This multistep approach allows the time needed to gather collateral information, such as ADHD rating scales completed by both teachers and family members for subsequent review.

When multiple problems are identified in an initial very brief appointment, working with a young person and his or her caregivers to jointly identify the leading problem allows for a more practical use of time. For instance, if a child is having screaming tantrums, is hitting other children, is sleeping poorly, and sometimes appears anxious, the identified leading problem may be the unsafe externalizing behaviors. In that case, the child's sleep problems and intermittent anxiety might be set aside to explore further at the next appointment.

Education About Mental Health Treatment

Educating children and families about their diagnosed mental health disorders has intrinsic value. Besides fulfilling an inherent desire to better understand problems, the ultimate purpose of providing psychoeducation is to increase the child's and his or her caregiver's ability to achieve health. Resistance to bringing a child to see a mental health practitioner or to trying out an appropriate psychiatric medication is common. So even if you make the best diagnosis possible, it does little good unless you connect the diagnosis to treatment. We keep the timeless advice of the physician Henry Cohen (1943) in mind: "All diagnoses are provisional formulae designed for action" (p. 24).

Therefore, we follow referral recommendations with educating the family about the value of receiving mental health services. This helps a patient and his or her caregivers visualize the process of treatment, what is known about the anticipated response to treatment, and what is likely to happen without treatment. For instance, we might help a caregiver with reluctance to see a mental health specialist understand that it takes an episode of untreated major depression a mean of about 8 months to self-resolve, which, if that happens, is a great deal of life and normal development for a child to miss out on (Birmaher et al. 2007). For a family who, because of the child's dysfunction, has lost some of their empathy for their child (which can happen with externalizing problems such as oppositional defiant disorder), providing blame-free psycho-education about the condition and the likelihood of response to treatment can also help can also help to reestablish caregiver empathy and support.

Teaching Patients and Caregivers Self-Help Strategies

Even though a primary care practitioner might prefer to have a mental health practitioner initiate all forms of intervention for an identified disorder, this delays care. Delays can occur from stigma-related resistance to following through on a referral, challenges in negotiating insurance restrictions, and having to wait for a local practitioner to become available. We prefer that some form of treatment plan initiation occur right away, through the kind of steps that would be appropriate for a family primary care practitioner to recommend.

What would be appropriate treatment to recommend without a mental health practitioner? The first step in treatment plan initiation could be coaching the child and family on self-help measures they can implement now. For example, the practitioner could address a young person's poor sleep habits, which accompany many different mental and behavioral health problems. Coaching how to improve a child's sleep hygiene, such as restricting access to text messaging after a certain time at night, can reduce daytime irritability and initiate improvements in mood, as we discuss in Chapter 14, "Psychosocial Interventions."

We also recommend a few situation-specific self-help readings or videos, which are known generically as *bibliotherapy*. Behavior management training for disruptive behavior is a prime example, because we know that a motivated parent can make significant changes in the child's discipline plan and environment from such references alone, without a therapist's involvement (Lavigne et al. 2008). Many high-quality books, Web sites, and videos are available that motivated parents can use to try implementing evidence-based disruptive behavior management or cognitive-behavior therapy informed skills. However, even when parents use high-quality self-help tools, this is less likely to make a difference with more severe symptoms, more overall family dysfunction, and more diagnostic complexity.

Initiation of Counseling and Therapy

We recommend psychotherapy for any young person who meets criteria for a mental health diagnosis with moderate to severe symptoms or for mild symptoms that are persistent and dysfunctional enough to warrant the investment of a young person's time. There are exceptions to this broad generalization about when to recommend psychotherapy; for instance, even in severe cases of ADHD, the young person may be treated successfully with medications alone, but this situation is an exception to the rule. The specific preferred forms of psychotherapy will differ by disorder type, so we encourage you to identify the diagnosis first and then consider the options we describe in Chapter 15, "Psychotherapeutic Interventions." Because many families avoid going to psychotherapy, you should learn their concerns and address them. For instance, *"You looked like you weren't very happy with the idea of working with a therapist...what comes to mind for you about this?"*

One-on-one psychotherapy is not the only source of outpatient services for young patients. Locally available support groups, crisis intervention services, parenting classes, social skills groups, family therapy, special education services, and speech therapists are just a few other examples. Because caregivers' own mental health difficulties may affect a young person's mental health disorders, coaching a caregiver on his or her own appropriate use of psychotherapy may be a way to help a child or an adolescent. Use of a question such as the following may help: *"With everything going on, do you have someone in your corner who is there just to help you?"* Some primary care practitioners may choose to provide young people with motivational interviewing techniques to support their efforts to reduce substance abuse behaviors or learn to provide coaching on relaxation training or other cognitive-behavioral techniques during their own follow-up appointments.

Appropriate Prescription of Medications

Primary care practitioners often feel pressured to prescribe right away, in part because the prescription pad is one of the few treatment tools immediately available. This can be quite appropriate when the diagnosis is clear, significant rather than just mild symptoms are present, an evidence-supported medication option is available, and the practitioner has discussed the risks and benefits. We otherwise advise resisting an immediate prescription.

A near-universal recommendation when prescribing psychiatric medications to children is that some form of psychosocial intervention—therapy or changes in the child's environment—should accompany their use. Other prescribing principles to keep in mind include starting with low doses and increasing slowly over time ("start low, go slow") and changing only one medication at a time to avoid outcomes confusion.

In summary, here are suggestions for a primary care approach to child mental health treatment:

- Instill appropriate hope, even in the initial interview.
- Form a therapeutic alliance with the young person and his caregivers.
- Use rating scales to help gather more clinical information but be aware of their limitations.
- Ask for collateral information from other informants to help ensure a correct diagnosis.
- Interview adolescents alone to obtain a more complete history, especially for internalizing disorders.
- Note the child's office behavior and interactions, which supply much of your child mental status examination findings.
- For an initial brief assessment, make only a provisional DSM-5 "unspecified" diagnosis.
- Expect to use more than one appointment to refine your diagnoses.
- Coach the family on pursuing their next best steps in care while screening for any barriers to address.
- For mild conditions, start with self-help approaches, bibliotherapy, and school interventions.
- Consider referring to specialist care anyone who is more ill or not improving.
- Use psychosocial interventions, such as psychotherapy, in most scenarios.
- If symptoms are moderate to severe, consider starting medication management with an evidence-supported strategy.
- Use your local specialists for support, to provide counseling, and to manage your more challenging patients.
- Schedule a follow-up appointment, even if patients were referred to specialty care.

Common Ages for Disorder Presentations

As we assess young people, we find it helpful to remember a maxim of clinical practice: "When you hear hoof beats, think horses, not zebras."

We find it to easier to detect psychiatric conditions in young people by recognizing the typical ages when different mental health conditions are likely to appear. For instance, you are unlikely to diagnose anorexia nervosa, bipolar disorder, or schizophrenia in a 4-year-old in a primary care clinic.

Still, there are not precise ages at which you should or should not consider a particular diagnosis. We can offer no firm rules. We can offer two pieces of prudent advice:

1. Remember the adage "Common things are common." When you are seeing a 10-year-old, separation anxiety disorder is more likely than schizophrenia.
2. Consider that developmental delay can influence the age and appearance of a disorder. For instance, encopresis, which is rarely seen in teenagers, may be more likely in a 16-year-old with the approximate mental age of a 4-year-old.

We created Table 2–1 to help guide your diagnostic inquiries. You will notice that as children age, conditions such as encopresis and oppositional defiant disorder become less likely, whereas conditions such as bipolar disorder and schizophrenia become more likely. Overall, diagnosable conditions increase with age. We advise against diagnosing personality disorders until at least late adolescence because, by definition, a child's personality is developing and changing more actively than is an adult's personality.

Another way to think of the predicted likelihood of detecting specific disorders in children is in regard to their absolute frequencies of occurrence. According to National Comorbidity Survey data (Merikangas et al. 2010), anxiety disorders have a much earlier age at onset than many practitioners realize. Half of individuals who develop an anxiety disorder will have had symptom onset by age 6, half of those with behavior disorders will have had onset by age 11, and half of those with mood disorders will have had onset by age 13 (among adolescents who have a mental health diagnosis). Table 2–2 includes the relative distribution of the lifetime experience of mental health diagnoses in decreasing overall order of frequency among 13- to 18-year-old patients in this survey.

Age-Based Behavioral Health Screening

Knowing when different mental and behavioral health disorders typically appear in young people can help your diagnostic process. Any screening test or diagnostic inquiry has more positive predictive value the higher the overall prevalence of the condition being investigated. Therefore, on the basis of prevalence rates and our own clinical experiences, the following are our suggestions for routine consideration in your differential diagnosis at different age ranges.

Ages 0–5: Developmental impairments and disruptive behavior problems are the predominant issues at this age. General screening rating scales to consider at this age therefore include general developmental assessments, autism spectrum screens, and social-emotional learning measures.

Ages 6–12: Attention-deficit/hyperactivity disorder (ADHD), disruptive, impulse-control, and conduct disorders; intellectual disabilities; anxiety disorders; and mood disorders predominate at this age. General screening rating scales to consider at this age therefore include ADHD symptom rating scales, anxiety rating scales, and depression and autism spectrum measures.

Ages 13–18: Major depressive disorder, anxiety disorders, posttraumatic stress disorder, eating disorders, ADHD, substance use disorder, and conduct disorder predominate at this age. General screening rating scales to consider at this age therefore include ADHD symptom rating scales, anxiety rating scales, and depression rating scales.

TABLE 2–1. Selected DSM-5 disorders to be considered at different ages

Preschool (2–5 years)	School age (6–12 years)	Adolescence (13–17 years)
ADHD (age ≥3, if severe)	ADHD	ADHD
Autism spectrum disorder	Adjustment disorder	Adjustment disorder
Communication disorders	Conduct disorder	Anorexia nervosa
Encopresis	Encopresis	Bipolar disorders
Intellectual disability (intellectual developmental disorder)	Intellectual disability (intellectual developmental disorder)	Bulimia
Oppositional defiant disorder	Insomnia disorder and parasomnias	Conduct disorder
Selective mutism	Specific learning disorder	Persistent depressive disorder (dysthymia)
Separation anxiety	Major depressive disorder	Intellectual disability (intellectual developmental disorder)
Specific phobia	Obsessive-compulsive disorder	Insomnia disorder
	Oppositional defiant disorder	Generalized anxiety disorder
	Posttraumatic stress disorder	Specific learning disorder
	Tourette's disorder (tics)	Major depressive disorder
	Trichotillomania (hair-picking disorder)	

TABLE 2–1. Selected DSM-5 disorders to be considered at different ages (*continued*)

Preschool (2–5 years)	School age (6–12 years)	Adolescence (13–17 years)
	Social anxiety disorder	Obstructive sleep apnea hypopnea
	Specific phobia	Obsessive-compulsive disorder
	Somatic symptom disorder	Oppositional defiant disorder
		Panic disorder
		Posttraumatic stress disorder
		Tourette's disorder (tics)
		Trichotillomania (hair-picking disorder)
		Schizophrenia
		Social anxiety disorder
		Specific phobia
		Somatic symptom disorder
		Substance use disorders

Note. ADHD=attention-deficit/hyperactivity disorder.
Source. American Psychiatric Association 2013.

TABLE 2–2. Cumulative prevalence of DSM-IV disorders in adolescents, per the National Comorbidity Survey–Adolescent Supplement

Disorder	Total prevalence (%)	Presence of severe impairment among those with disorder (%)
Specific phobia	19.3	3
Oppositional defiant disorder	12.6	52
Major depressive disorder or dysthymia	11.7	74
Social phobia	9.1	17
Drug abuse or dependence	8.9	NR
Attention-deficit/ hyperactivity disorder	8.7	8
Separation anxiety disorder	7.6	8
Conduct disorder	6.8	32
Alcohol abuse or dependence	6.4	NR
Posttraumatic stress disorder	5.0	30
Bipolar disorder	2.9	89
Eating disorder	2.7	NR
Agoraphobia	2.4	100
Panic disorder	2.3	100
Generalized anxiety disorder	2.2	41

Note.   NR=not reported.
Source.   Derived from Merikangas et al. 2010.

Chapter 3

Common Clinical Concerns

Although every child or adolescent is unique, a handful of common concerns account for most of the reasons young people come to clinical attention. You learn to recognize these patterns during training. You see hundreds of children and adolescents, discuss them with clinical supervisors, and develop a subconscious ability to quickly recognize the ways a particular child resembles common concerning patterns. For instance, you may quickly recognize a child's presentation pattern as typical of an uncomplicated adjustment to a new school rather than an episode of major depression. These subconscious patterns are a tremendous benefit to a practitioner because they help her improve her clinical efficiency.

However, relying on experience to guide your current practice causes at least two problems.

First, even seasoned practitioners make mistakes. We assume that an adolescent has an ordinary case of unhappiness, so we neglect to consider whether her social isolation is the result of abuse or psychosis. We assume that a child's inability to play well with others represents a neurodevelopmental disorder, so we neglect to ask about cultural expectations for interactive play in a family. Even an experienced practitioner needs to remain curious about a particular patient and vigilant about the eventuality of making mistakes.

Second, most young people are evaluated and treated for mental illness by primary care practitioners with limited mental health training. These practitioners often have remarkable stores of clinical experience in caring for children and adolescents, but their mental health training is often limited to a few afternoons, a long-ago clinical rotation, or an occasional lecture. A practitioner whose training is not specialized for mental health can benefit from referencing prudent aids to decision making.

The following sections, and their accompanying tables, are prudent guides to common clinical concerns. Each table identifies a common clinical concern, provides diagnostic categories to which these concerns can be mapped, and suggests questions to guide clinical inquiry. We designed most questions to be asked of a young person. When a question is designed to be asked of a caregiver, we label it "for caregiver."

Poor Academic Performance

To succeed in a work environment, a person needs the ability to succeed, the desire to succeed, and an environment that enables success. Major life distractions or impairing illnesses can unfortunately derail a person who would have otherwise found success. Although that simple description can be used to describe just about any adult workplace, the exact same points are true about children in school. School is where children and adolescents go to work.

When you see a child who is struggling to succeed in school, it is useful to think very broadly about what might be getting in her way (Table 3–1). Just like an adult who is having workplace difficulties, a young person may have problems with 1) ability, 2) desire or effort, 3) work environment, 4) life distraction, or 5) an impairing mental health disorder or illness.

1. *Ability* challenges we consider right away to ensure we do not miss them. The most basic ability is our senses. Hearing and vision screens are easy to perform, and when needed, an intervention such as a hearing aid or a new pair of glasses can make a profound difference. Motor impairments, such as the physical ability to write or enunciate clearly, also can be managed effectively through physical, occupational, or speech therapy.

   Intellectual disabilities, of course, influence school success. You can determine whether a young child has fallen behind on developmental milestones by comparing her traits with a list of normal range expectations. Caregiver-completed developmental rating scale measures such as the Ages & Stages Questionnaires (ASQ) will aid this task, or you can simply ask a caregiver if she has had any concerns about the child's speech, comprehension, or physical ability development. We would suspect an intellectual disability when the child has multiple areas of delay. IQ test scores provide helpful

TABLE 3–1. Poor academic performance

Diagnostic category	Suggested screening questions
First consider	
Abuse	*"Has anything or anyone made you feel uncomfortable or unsafe?"* (for caregiver) *"Has anything happened to your child that really shouldn't have happened?"*
Bullying	*"Have other kids been teasing you or making you feel afraid?"*
Sensory impairment	*"Have you ever noticed any trouble with hearing or vision?"*
Common diagnostic possibilities	
Attention-deficit/ hyperactivity disorder	(for caregiver) *"Even when she wants to learn, is your child too inattentive or hyperactive to succeed?"*
Intellectual disability (intellectual developmental disorder)	(for caregiver) *"Have there always been problems with learning? Were there early milestone delays such as speech delays?"*
Specific learning disorder	*"Are any specific subjects or activities such as reading particularly difficult?"*
Mood or anxiety disorder	(for caregiver) *"Did poor school performance come after an anxious or depressive change?"*
Oppositional defiant disorder or conduct disorder	(for caregiver) *"Is your child simply refusing to do schoolwork?"*
Substance use disorder	*"Have you been using drugs or alcohol?"*

data, but impairments in adaptive life functioning also must be present to diagnose an intellectual disability. Early intervention services or a local school district's special education program should be engaged as early as possible to improve outcomes when global developmental delay or an intellectual disability is suspected.

Specific learning disabilities are often detected much later than a general intellectual disability because they may not become apparent until school demands increase. The three overall categories of specific learning disabilities are reading, writing, and computation. The hallmark of a specific learning disability is that the child has an area of much poorer school performance than expected on the basis of the child's overall intellect and effort.

2. *Desire or effort* in school is about the motivation to achieve. A person with a low to average intellect but a strong motivation to achieve can have greater school success than someone with high intellect but low motivation to achieve. There is no quick fix for motivation problems. For young children, motivation in school starts with healthy home relationships and regularly experienced positive parent-child time, which foster a desire to meet adult expectations. Clear and reasonable family expectations for the child's school achievement are also necessary. For older children, this desire ideally evolves into working hard in school because they want to please themselves.

3. *Work environment* affects performance because not every school and not every classroom will suit every child. For instance, an easily distracted child will not do well in a loud and overcrowded classroom, and a child with a specific writing disability will not do well in a class that requires large volumes of daily written work completion. Asking about the class environment and the child's home workspace may identify these issues.

4. *Life distractions* prevent success by taking a child's mind off his or her schoolwork. Abuse, neglect, and bullying are the most important distractions for us to catch right away so that child protective services or school officials can intervene. Children may experience a decline in school performance because of family stressors such as parental separation or divorce or from struggling with peer relationships. It is useful to ask, *"When you try to do your schoolwork but get distracted, what's on your mind?"*

5. *Impairing mental health disorders or illnesses* that are described in DSM-5 (American Psychiatric Association 2013) can create school problems. For instance, major depressive disorder, persistent depressive disorder (dysthymia), generalized anxiety disorder (GAD), obsessive-compulsive disorder (OCD), social anxiety disorder (social phobia), oppositional defiant disorder (ODD), conduct disorder, substance use disorder, and posttraumatic stress disorder (PTSD) all will reduce a child's school performance. Chronic medical diseases, especially those that involve experiencing daily pain, also will reduce the ability to focus on school.

Attention-deficit/hyperactivity disorder (ADHD) is the main mental disorder that gets considered in terms of a high overall incidence (>5%) and common family requests for treatment. We would look for ADHD if attention and/or hyperactivity-related schooling difficulties can be traced back to the early elementary school years and these difficulties are not readily attributed to any of the above causes. Sudden-onset attention problems are thus unlikely to be caused by ADHD. Another key trait to look for is whether ADHD-like symptoms are present in multiple settings (such as both in school and at home). The good news is that by correctly identifying an impairing illness such as ADHD, you have an opportunity to treat and resolve the schooling problem.

Developmental Delay

A person's development from infancy to adulthood is amazing in its breadth and complexity. Because not every person develops at the same pace or in the same order of skill acquisition, detecting a significant developmental impairment may be challenging (Table 3–2). For instance, a child may learn to walk without ever crawling or may appear speech delayed at 18 months but speech advanced at 2 years. Fewer than half of the children with significant developmental delays are identified before starting school, which delays entry into treatment. Therefore, anything practitioners can do to help caregivers detect these problems can alter the trajectory of a child's life. A key function of health maintenance care in the first 5 years of life is to detect developmental impairments that would benefit from an intervention. Any parental concerns expressed about a child's speech, learning, sociability,

TABLE 3–2. Developmental delay

Diagnostic category	Suggested screening questions for caregiver
First consider	
Neurodegenerative conditions	*"Has your child lost any previously acquired skills or abilities?"*
Sensory impairment	*"Have you ever noticed any trouble with your child's hearing or vision?"*
Common diagnostic possibilities	
Autism spectrum disorder	*"Does your child smile in response to your smile? Did your child respond to her own name before age 1? Does your child have restricted interests or behaviors?"*
Communication disorder	*"Does your child have problems with stuttering or with understanding words?"*
Fragile X syndrome	*"Does your child have siblings or relatives on the mother's side of the family with intellectual impairment?"*
Intellectual disability (intellectual developmental disorder) or global developmental delay	*"Was your child slow to develop speech and physical skills? Does your child have a harder time learning new things than other children?"*
Neurobehavioral disorder associated with prenatal alcohol exposure	*"What can you tell me about alcohol use during pregnancy? Has your child had difficulty regulating his or her mood or impulses?"*

or physical skills should open the proverbial door for further examination.

Development can be broken down into three broad categories: cognitive, motor, and social-emotional. *Cognitive development* refers to what most people think of as intelligence. Some measurable areas of cognition include problem solving, language, memory, information processing, and attention. *Motor development* refers to the acquisition of gross motor (e.g., run, throw) and fine motor (e.g., pincer grasp, drawing) physical motion skills. *Social-emotional development* refers to the acquisition of the ability to interact with others and manage the emotions of social interactions.

Because there is a very wide range of what can be considered "normal" development, we look for developmental markers that are far enough outside the norm to justify referral for developmental assessments or interventions. When parents express that they already have concerns about a specific area of their child's development, we will likely find a need for a developmental assessment referral. Speech therapists can help with suspected communication delays, physical therapists can help with suspected motor skill delays, and special education–sponsored preschools can help with suspected socialization and general learning skill delays. All children with significant developmental delays should be referred to early intervention services.

Detecting autism spectrum disorder before a child reaches age 3 years is aided by recognizing certain red flags in social-emotional development. These include not smiling in response to being smiled at, not making eye contact, not sharing attention with others, not responding to her own name by age 1 year, poor social interest, and a lack of interest in other children. Socially focused interventions that foster communication as early as possible are a cornerstone of autism care.

Every child with developmental impairment should be screened for hearing or vision impairments because sensory impairments can worsen or even cause developmental impairments. Another reason for early sensory assessments is that hearing and vision impairments can be relatively easy to treat.

A developmental impairment rarely worsens over time, so when we find any loss of previously acquired skills, we broaden our search for an etiology to include medical causes. For example, hypothyroidism, phenylketonuria, and recurrent seizures are some of the many medical causes of regressing development.

We recommend considering genetic testing if the clinical pattern might fit a genetic disorder. For instance, fragile X testing is particularly pertinent if other family members have intellectual disability. If no specific genetic disorder is suspected, the yield of genetic testing will be reduced. Developmental disorder laboratory tests for fragile X and chromosome microarray should be ordered only after providing pretest counseling to families. Family risks from genetic testing include finding an unknown significance mutation that creates more anxiety than answers or learning something the family did not wish to learn, such as misattributed paternity or a pessimistic prognosis that lowers current quality of life.

Diagnosing a child with neurobehavioral disorder associated with prenatal alcohol exposure, included in Section III of DSM-5, can be a challenge to your therapeutic alliance with caregivers because it inherently assigns blame for some of a child's problems on her mother's behaviors during pregnancy. Characteristic facial features (thin upper lip, smooth philtrum, short palpebral fissure length) might be present, but their absence does not rule out the diagnosis. Because these children do have a unique prognosis, it is worth exploring this possibility in a blame-free fashion.

In Chapter 12, "Developmental Milestones," we further review developmental milestones and discuss developmental red flags, signs that need further evaluation, ideally through specialized developmental assessments.

Disruptive or Aggressive Behavior

When we see a young person who is aggressive or disruptive, we receive that behavior as a form of communication. A child who is unable to effectively communicate verbally may use behaviors instead, such as lashing out at a peer who has just taken her toy. Hunger, pain, sadness, fear, and frustration are just a few examples of distress that may turn into tantrums, disruptive behavior, or aggression. For instance, if you can identify that hunger leads to a tantrum in a nonverbal child, the child can be coached to point at a picture of food to communicate hunger and get something to eat (this is known as a *picture exchange system*).

A *functional analysis of behavior* is an overall approach that helps with most aggression problems in childhood. In a functional analysis, you identify the character, timing, frequency, and duration of at least a few incidents of disruptive, aggressive behavior in great detail. Predisposing, precipitating, and perpetuating influences on behavior can be elicited by asking a series of questions such as *"Tell me about the last time this happened. What was happening right before? How had that day been going overall? What did you do while the behavior was happening? What happened right afterward?"*

What you often discover from the unedited details of two or three incidents is that the aggressive and disruptive behaviors begin to make a lot more sense. Examples include tantrums inadvertently being rewarded with treats because caregivers want the child to stop in the moment or aggression that allows a child to successfully escape aversive situations.

Different DSM-5 disorders may be suggested by particular circumstances of the child's disruptive behaviors (Table 3–3). Children with PTSD may become disruptive when situations remind them of past negative events. Children with a learning disability may be disruptive when struggling at school or working on homework. A child with ADHD may have nearly continuous, disruptive hyperactivity that is not situational or vindictive. A child with social anxiety disorder (social phobia) or autism spectrum disorder may show disruptive behavior when pushed to engage in social situations. A child who has been bullied at school may suddenly develop disruptive, lashing-out behavior or become resistant to going to school. In summary, identifying the overall pattern and context of behaviors is key to the diagnostic process.

It is relatively easy to identify ODD, a diagnosis that describes pervasively negativistic and defiant behavior toward authority figures in a developmentally inappropriate fashion (i.e., not just the "terrible twos") that lasts for more than 6 months. The real challenge is knowing what to do about it.

ODD has a complex, multifactorial etiology. In simple terms, ODD represents a mismatch in fit between a child's inherent traits or temperament and how her caregivers and authority figures respond to them. Communicating to caregivers that they share responsibility with their child for the negative behavior patterns in ODD without this being perceived as blaming them for the problem is a tricky balance. One way to do so is to characterize the child's personality or biology as requiring higher-than-usual parenting demands, so more highly skilled parenting strategies are needed to respond to ODD. Empathy for the challenge parents face goes a long way here.

TABLE 3–3. Disruptive or aggressive behavior

Diagnostic category	Suggested screening questions
First consider	
Abuse	*"Has anything or anyone made you feel uncomfortable or unsafe?"* (for caregiver) *"Has anything happened to your child that really shouldn't have happened?"*
Bullying	*"Have other kids been teasing you or making you feel afraid?"*
Safety	*"Have you been thinking about or planning to hurt anyone?"*
Common diagnostic possibilities	
Attention-deficit/ hyperactivity disorder	(for caregiver) *"Does your child consistently have trouble paying attention, or is she hyperactive or disruptive?"*
Communication disorder	(for caregiver) *"Is your child aggressive when she has needs she cannot communicate?"*
Conduct disorder	(for caregiver) *"Has your child been committing serious violations of rules and the rights of others for more than a year?"*
Oppositional defiant disorder	(for caregiver) *"Has your child been unusually defiant and oppositional for more than 6 months?"*
Posttraumatic stress disorder	(for caregiver) *"Does your child's disruptive behavior primarily occur after reminders or memories of past trauma?"*

Conduct disorder is a similar, but more concerning, version of defiant, aggressive behavior that has a greater risk of continuing into adulthood. Conduct disorder should be suspected when a child is committing serious violations of the rights of others, such as stealing, initiating fights, using a weapon to threaten others, destroying property, or running away from home.

Successful management of ODD and conduct disorder requires motivating authority figures in a child's environment to make changes in how they interact with the child. The traditional one-on-one psychotherapy approach rarely will be sufficient. Behavior management training is the best overall treatment strategy for both ODD and conduct disorder. There are many types of behavior management training, but they all share a focus on coaching parents and caregivers to set better limits and expectations for the child and a focus on the child and parents regularly spending positive times together, thus providing opportunities for the child to experience praise. Historically, this approach was referred to as *parent training*, but we think that term should be discarded for unnecessarily assigning fault to the parents, which reduces the therapeutic alliance and motivation for change. The more severe the symptoms, the more community inclusive the behavior management approach should be, such as how multisystemic therapy also engages nonparental authority figures in the community for patients with conduct disorder.

Medications are generally not the preferred treatment for disruptive or aggressive behavior. However, if the child has a specific DSM-5 diagnosis that is known to be medication responsive, such as ADHD or major depressive disorder, then medication treatment typically will improve disruptive or aggressive behavior. No medications are indicated for the treatment of ODD or conduct disorder, whose best treatment is via coaching and supporting the child's authority figures. If a disruptive or aggressive problem is considered to be highly impairing and other appropriate interventions have been tried and have failed, then a nonspecific medication to diminish maladaptive or impulsive aggression may be considered. If this is done, we would recommend a clonidine or guanfacine trial first because if they are helpful, their use presents few long-term medical risks. Second-generation antipsychotics such as risperidone may be effective in reducing aggression, but antipsychotics have more significant adverse effects and should be reserved for the most severe scenarios (Loy et al. 2012).

Withdrawn or Sad Mood

When a young person presents as withdrawn or sad (Table 3–4), we always assess for the presence of a major depressive episode. Two or more weeks of depressed or irritable mood, along with multiple neurovegetative symptoms (decreased energy, concentration, interest, or physical activity; thoughts of self-harm; changes in appetite or sleep; and feelings of guilt or worthlessness), would suggest a major depressive episode. In contrast, persistent depressive disorder (dysthymia) is essentially a low-grade depression that has been present for more than a year in a child, without relief for more than 2 months during that time. If the sad mood was triggered by a stressful event within the past 3 months and neither major depression nor dysthymia is diagnosable, an adjustment disorder with depressed mood may be present.

Regardless of whether a withdrawn or sad child has an active mood disorder, routinely asking about self-harm risks is important. Adolescents may see even a single disappointment—such as a relationship breakup—as so catastrophic that they feel suicidal or begin to hurt themselves. This means that as practitioners we must ask about suicidal thoughts and self-harm urges even if we believe that a young person is experiencing only a time-limited adjustment disorder. With practice, we find that asking about suicidality and self-harm comes as naturally as asking any other question. It helps to keep in mind that asking about suicidal thoughts does not create a risk of self-harm. Instead, it reduces risks by showing you care.

Although medically induced depression is uncommon in a young person, all practitioners must be alert to the possibility. For instance, testing for hypothyroidism is reasonable if a patient experienced physical symptoms such as fatigue before mood changes developed. Because anemia is a common problem in young people, a complete blood count should be considered to assess its presence in a patient who is fatigued. Iatrogenic origins of depression should be considered as well, such as when a child starting β-blockers or isotretinoin subsequently experiences dysphoria.

Recurrent substance abuse can cause an adolescent to appear depressed. Because we find that adolescents typically assert that they see their substance use as helping their mood, establishing a timeline of what came first may help you con-

TABLE 3–4. Withdrawn or sad mood

Diagnostic category	Suggested screening questions
First consider	
Abuse	*"Has anything or anyone made you feel uncomfortable or unsafe?"* (for caregiver) *"Has anything happened to your child that really shouldn't have happened?"*
Bullying	*"Have other kids been teasing you or making you feel afraid?"*
Medical conditions (anemia, hypothyroidism)	*"Did all of your symptoms seem to start with fatigue?"*
Self-harm	*"Have you been thinking about hurting yourself? Have you ever hurt yourself or attempted suicide? Do you have any plans to hurt yourself?"*
Common diagnostic possibilities	
Adjustment disorder with depressed mood	*"Did your sad or down mood start right after a stressful event in the past few months?"*
Bipolar disorder	*"Has there ever been a period of multiple days in a row when you were the opposite of depressed, with very high energy and little need for sleep? If so, can you tell me more about that time?"*
Persistent depressive disorder (dysthymia)	*"Have you been sad or gloomy most days of the week for more than a year?"*
Major depressive disorder	*"Have you felt really down, depressed, or uninterested in things you used to enjoy for more than 2 weeks?"*
Substance use disorder	*"Have you been using drugs or alcohol?"*

vince your patient to discontinue the substance at least temporarily and find out how she feels after a few weeks of being substance free.

Bipolar disorder is relatively uncommon in children but should be considered. To detect the possibility of bipolar depression, we ask caregivers if the child has ever had a history of discrete mood elevation and energy increase of multiple days' duration with accompanying manic symptoms (e.g., racing thoughts or speech, unusual risk taking, and decreased need for sleep). Notably, the presence of an irritable mood is not a reliable indicator of bipolar disorder in children. If you suspect that a young person with a withdrawn or sad mood has bipolar disorder, monotherapy with antidepressants should be avoided because of their risk for inducing a manic episode.

Every child with a moderate to severe depressive disorder should be referred for an evidence-based psychotherapy, such as cognitive-behavioral therapy (CBT) or interpersonal therapy. Because the level of family motivation to use psychotherapy is a common problem, we often address this up front by informing families that psychotherapy is the most effective strategy available to reduce the risks of suicidality. Caregivers of a young person can also take the safety steps of restricting impulsive access to firearms and dangerous pills and maintaining increased awareness and monitoring. In the presence of active suicide plans or the inability to maintain immediate safety, practitioners should consider admission to a crisis stabilization unit, day treatment program, or psychiatric inpatient treatment. Families also can help the child by promoting "behavioral activation" treatment for depression at home through scheduling desirable exercise and social activities.

The current view on selective serotonin reuptake inhibitor (SSRI) use for depression is that some young patients might experience an increase in suicidal thoughts during the first few months of SSRI use, but most do not, and overall, the benefits of use outweigh potential risks for a moderate to severe depression. A prudent practitioner will warn patients about the possible risk, stay connected with patients and the patient's caregivers after the initial prescription to inquire specifically about increased irritability or suicidal thoughts at least twice in the first month of use, and strongly consider stopping the medication should increased irritability or suicidality occur (Bridge et al. 2007).

Because of its large research evidence base indicating benefits in young people, fluoxetine is widely considered the first-line choice for adolescent major depressive disorder. Second-line SSRI choices based on the evidence include sertraline and escitalopram or citalopram. Usual adolescent depression starting doses are 10 mg for fluoxetine, 25–50 mg for sertraline, 10 mg for citalopram, and 5 mg for escitalopram; about half of these amounts are used in preadolescents. Doses should be increased after 4–6 weeks if the medications are well tolerated but have insufficient benefits. SSRIs are most effective when used in combination with psychotherapy, which is another reason to promote the family's engagement with psychotherapy. Persistent depressive disorder (dysthymia) would be treated with the same medications but is notably slower to respond (McVoy and Findling 2013).

Irritable or Labile Mood

A young person may experience an irritable or labile mood for several reasons (Table 3–5). Several mental disorders—bipolar disorders, depressive disorders, anxiety disorders, PTSD, and ODD—should be considered because irritability can be a symptom of a mental disorder. It also can be a symptom of substance abuse, a reaction to challenging life situations or maltreatment, or a normal variation in mood. When irritability is the primary complaint, we counsel a broad search for clues as to "why."

Unfortunately, there has been a major misdiagnosis problem during the past two decades because chronically irritable, labile moods in children were being interpreted as being pathognomonic of a childhood bipolar disorder. This was usually incorrect, in that few (if any) chronically irritable children were later found to have bipolar disorder as young adults (Birmaher et al. 2014). Unless a child has multiday duration manic symptoms occurring during a discrete episode that represents a break from baseline functioning, we counsel against diagnosing bipolar disorder in children and adolescents.

In part because of this perceived need to have a diagnosis that better characterizes children with life dysfunction because of chronically irritable moods, a new diagnosis was created. Disruptive mood dysregulation disorder is a new DSM-5 diagnosis for children who have more than a year of

TABLE 3–5. Irritable or labile mood

Diagnostic category	Suggested screening questions
First consider	
Abuse	"Has anything or anyone made you feel uncomfortable or unsafe?" (for caregiver) "Has anything happened to your child that really shouldn't have happened?"
Substance abuse	"Have you been using drugs or alcohol?"
Suicidality	"Have you had thoughts about hurting yourself?"
Common diagnostic possibilities	
Bipolar disorder	"Has there ever been a period of multiple days in a row when you were the opposite of depressed, with super high energy and little need for sleep? If so, can you tell me more about that time?"
Disruptive mood dysregulation disorder	(for caregiver) "Has your child had severe and persistent irritability along with frequent temper outbursts?"
Major depressive disorder	"Have you felt really down, depressed, or uninterested in things you used to enjoy for more than 2 weeks?"
Oppositional defiant disorder	(for caregiver) "Has your child been unusually defiant and oppositional for more than 6 months?"
Posttraumatic stress disorder	(for caregiver) "Does the irritability or moodiness worsen after reminders or memories of past trauma?"

significant daily dysphoric mood symptoms and temper out-bursts three or more times a week that are not better ex-plained by other conditions. However, this is a new diagnosis, so we know very little about prognosis or best treatments (Roy et al. 2014). Practically speaking, we believe disruptive mood dysregulation disorder could be considered as a variant of ODD in which mood symptoms predominate.

Even if a young person's irritability cannot ultimately be traced to a specific DSM-5 diagnosis with a known treatment, a generalized approach to managing irritable moods can still be helpful. We recommend enhancing family supports and providing behavior management training as appropriate for most types of irritable mood care. Creating calm, consistent, and caring limits and expectations within the household will typically improve behavior problems and irritability from a wide variety of causes.

Families with significant internal conflict can benefit from family therapy or from caregivers seeking their own individual supports. You may be able to motivate parents who report feeling exasperated with a child by using a "put your own mask on first" analogy, as with airline travel. An unnurtured parent who receives individual supports or professional help may greatly improve interactions with her child. For those children who are found to lack positive experiences with their caregivers, creating opportunities for praise and positive attention is a key to treatment success.

One-on-one counseling therapy is indicated for all mood disorders and anxiety-related conditions (including PTSD) with an irritability component. Medication is never indicated for irritable mood without a specific diagnosis.

Anxious or Avoidant Behavior

When a child is struggling with being worried or anxious, we first check if something in a child's world is directly causing this feeling. Anxiety from being bullied, from experiencing a major traumatic event, or from living in an abusive household should appropriately generate self-protective avoidance behaviors. Only after we know that no realistic threat to the child exists and have determined that the child's anxiety causes significant life dysfunction do we consider an anxiety disorder diagnosis (Table 3–6).

TABLE 3–6. Anxious or avoidant behavior

Diagnostic category	Suggested screening questions
First consider	
Abuse	*"Has anything or anyone made you feel uncomfortable or unsafe?"* (for caregiver) *"Has anything happened to your child that really shouldn't have happened?"*
Bullying	*"Have other kids been teasing you or making you feel afraid?"*
Trauma	*"Have you been hurt recently or been in any accidents?"*
Self-harm	*"When you feel overwhelmed, do you think about hurting yourself?"*
Common diagnostic possibilities	
Generalized anxiety disorder	*"Do you feel tense, restless, or worried most of the time? Do these worries affect your sleep or performance at school?"*
Obsessive-compulsive disorder	*"Do you frequently have unwanted thoughts, images, or urges in your mind? Do you check or clean things to avoid those unwanted thoughts?"*
Panic disorder	*"Do you get sudden surges of fear that make your body feel shaky or your heart race? Do you change what you do in order to avoid having a panic experience?"*
Posttraumatic stress disorder	*"Do you startle easily or have frequent nightmares? Do you avoid reminders of traumatic events in your past?"* (for caregiver) *"Does the irritability or moodiness worsen after reminders or memories of past trauma?"*
Separation anxiety disorder	*"Is it hard to leave your house or hard to leave your mom or dad because of worries?"*
Specific phobia	*"Is there something in particular or a situation that makes you immediately afraid?"*

Children have worries during the course of their normal development, such as fears of strangers, separation, injury, or failure. Learning how to cope with anxious feelings by facing them directly is an important developmental task that, once mastered, enables future achievements. Parental anxiety may interfere with this process if it reinforces a child's fears or encourages avoidance behavior. For instance, inadvertent parental reinforcement of normal separation anxiety may turn this problem into a disorder unless the parent is taught more helpful strategies.

Children who feel anxious often struggle to find words to express how they feel. A child reporting stomachaches, nausea, chest pain, fatigue, or headaches may be functionally disclosing that she feels anxious, but through a biological mechanism such as autonomic nerves altering intestinal motility or arterial smooth muscle tone. In fact, the chief complaint of children and adolescents seeking mental health treatment in primary care settings often will be a physical ailment. When listening alertly for any meaning behind a physical ailment, practitioners should think about timing. Severe stomach cramps before attending school or headaches before performing in a sporting event will help identify anxiety disorders.

Common anxiety disorders for children include GAD, panic disorder, specific phobia, and separation anxiety disorder. These conditions could appear in a developmental trajectory, such as separation anxiety disorder during the elementary school years being replaced by specific phobias in middle school and then a GAD in the adolescent years. For some children, their anxiety trait persists, but the expressed form of that anxiety varies over time. Isolated panic attacks are a short-term anxiety symptom that may appear with other disorders such as depression. Panic disorder is different, involving a disabling fear of experiencing future panic episodes.

Anxiety disorders commonly run in families; thus, when a child is given an anxiety disorder diagnosis, either or both parents likely have struggled with anxiety disorders themselves. This familial tendency can occur through shared genetic traits, through children absorbing the anxious sentiments a parent generates within the household, or both. In some situations, the most effective way to help an anxious child is to help her parent to more effectively manage her own anxiety and thus create a more stable and supportive home environment for the child.

Strategies shown to be effective for anxiety treatment in children include different forms of psychotherapy in which exposure to feared thoughts or ideas is their most common element (Chorpita and Daleiden 2009). Repeated exposure to feared situations or memories that do not have any negative consequences, through repetition and reframing, will help the child's mind to unlearn that fear. However, if that fear is still a "real" one, such as a traumatized child at risk for future abuse, then psychotherapy alone will not be as beneficial until the child's safety is secured. CBT is the most commonly available modality for anxiety treatment that uses exposure.

Parents also must challenge or restrict the avoidance behaviors in their child because avoidance of a feared situation leads to a temporary relief of anxiety that over time reinforces the fear and worsens the severity of the anxiety. For instance, a fear of attending school becomes stronger if the child is allowed to repeatedly skip school. SSRIs, including sertraline and fluoxetine, have been shown in multiple studies to be effective in treating different forms of childhood anxiety disorders and are most effective when used in combination with psychotherapy (Mohatt et al. 2014).

OCD and PTSD are anxiety-related diagnoses that are now listed in their own sections of DSM-5: "Obsessive-Compulsive and Related Disorders" (which includes hoarding disorder and trichotillomania) and "Trauma- and Stressor-Related Disorders" (which includes acute stress and adjustment disorders). OCD responds very well to the same first-line therapies as used for other anxiety disorders: CBT and SSRIs. PTSD has been found to respond well to exposure-based therapies such as trauma-focused CBT, but its response to medications in children is not so well established.

Recurrent and Excessive Physical Complaints

Primary care practitioners know that recurrent headaches, chest pain, nausea, and fatigue are the presenting concern in about 10% of all office visits by adolescents, and recurrent abdominal pain alone is the presenting concern for about 5% of all pediatric office visits (Silber 2011). Although these somatic complaints may have many etiologies, the most common etiologies are psychiatric. Knowing this, whenever we hear a psychosomatic complaint, we consider whether anxiety disorders, depressive disorders, or adjustment disorders are the cause. Treatments for anxiety and depression are both effective and straightforward. The treatments for somatic disorders (somatic symptom disorder, factitious disorder, conversion disorder) are more challenging, so we consider them after ruling out anxiety and depressive disorders (Table 3–7).

We do not, however, favor considering somatic disorders only after excluding all possible causes for somatic complaints. Contemporary medicine overvalues biological explanations for somatic symptoms and usually leaves other explanations, including psychiatric etiologies, as diagnoses of exclusion. The unfortunate effects of a medical-before-psychiatric approach are that

- Mental illness may go unrecognized.
- Patients and parents may react poorly to hearing an "it is all in your head" explanation after multiple investigations and appointments.
- Families may try to prove that symptoms are "real" and insist on inappropriate tests or procedures.
- Acceptance of psychiatric care or forms of appropriate functional assistance may be decreased.

To counteract these pitfalls, we recommend describing psychiatric etiologies to families when presenting your *initial* somatic symptom differential diagnosis and then openly discussing them throughout. You can do this by describing what you think are the most likely psychobiological pathways for somatic symptoms. For instance, you can explain how stress affects the autonomic nervous system, which can lower gastric pH and alter intestinal motility (for nausea and abdominal pain) or can alter blood vessel smooth muscle tone (for headaches). By offering a biological account for physical symptoms of a mental illness, you will help patients and their caregivers more readily accept psychiatric interventions such as CBT and relaxation therapy because you have taught them that psychiatric intervention can modify autonomic nervous system functioning.

Children with somatic symptom disorders usually lack awareness that stress or anxiety is linked to their physical experiences or may lack an ability to adequately use words to describe their emotional states (referred to as *alexithymia*). The classic childhood pattern is that somatic symptoms increase before stressful experiences, such as attending school, visiting someone else's home, or performing publicly, whereas

TABLE 3–7. Recurrent and excessive physical complaints

Diagnostic category	Suggested screening questions
First consider	
Abuse or maltreatment	*"Has anything or anyone made you feel uncomfortable or unsafe?"* (for caregiver) *"Has anything happened to your child that really shouldn't have happened?"*
Adjustment disorder	*"Was there something stressful in the past 3 months that happened right before these symptoms appeared?"*
Anxiety disorders	(for caregiver) *"Does your child have a lot of worries that cause distress?"*
Depressive disorders	(for caregiver) *"Has your child's mood been unusually down or low for more than a couple of weeks?"*
Other diagnostic possibilities	
Conversion disorder	For practitioner: consider when you identify a loss of motor or sensory function that is inconsistent with recognized disorders.
Factitious disorder imposed on self	(for caregiver—asked away from the child) *"Do you suspect your child may be intentionally exaggerating symptoms?"*
Factitious disorder imposed on another	For practitioner: consider when parent has pattern of reporting symptoms in her child inconsistent with recognized disorders.
Panic attacks	*"Do you experience sudden surges of fear that make your body feel shaky or your heart race?"*
Somatic symptom disorder	(for caregiver) *"Does your child have recurrent physical symptoms that disrupt his or her daily life? Does your child have an excessive focus on his or her physical symptoms?"*

the somatic symptoms decrease if stressful situations are avoided. Specifically experienced symptoms may change over time, in that a child with recurrent abdominal pain early in life may develop recurrent headaches and fatigue as a teenager.

In the case of a conversion disorder with prominent unusual motor problems (such as paralysis of only one shoulder) or sensory problems (such as a loss of all feeling in the legs with normal reflexes), we similarly find it important to help the child exit her presentation without accusing her of having biologically "false" symptoms. For instance, you can explain to a patient that your examination identified no major medical difficulties but that in your experience other young people with similar symptoms experienced a fairly rapid resolution. A face-saving explanation such as "*I believe that in a short time your nerves will simply reset themselves, like how the seasons change*" may be particularly helpful. Successfully responding to conversion symptoms relies as much on the art of medicine as on the science of medicine.

A young person also may intentionally falsify symptoms to malinger when there is a clear secondary gain or as part of a factitious disorder. Detecting a case of factitious disorder imposed on another requires a practitioner to mentally shift his or her thinking to consider this possibility because it is difficult to accept that a caregiver might misrepresent, simulate, or cause signs of illness in her children. Suspected cases of factitious disorder are best managed by all of a patient's practitioners communicating directly with one another about their concerns, consulting local experts in this topic, and then arriving at a unified rather than divided approach to helping the child.

Sleep Problems

Sleep problems are very common, present in 5%–20% of children (Meltzer et al. 2010). Most childhood insomnia can be traced to poor sleep habits and inadequate enforcement of bedtime habits by caregivers. The contemporary incorporation of electronics into every aspect of daily life means that it is no longer sufficient for practitioners to simply recommend no television in the bedroom of a child with insomnia. Cell phones have effectively become sleep prevention devices through the applications, text messaging, and games they bring into the bedroom. Restricting all computer access and video game use after a certain time in the evening can yield a dramatic improvement in the amount of sleep that children (and their caregivers!) get.

Another key sleep hygiene problem is a loss of the behavioral association that being in bed equals sleep time. Behavioral routines around going to bed help signal to the brain when it is time to disconnect. Doing homework in bed, eating in bed, playing in bed, and communicating with friends from bed break that behavioral association. For those with insomnia, the act of lying awake in bed for a long time, staring at the clock, and waiting for sleep can become another sleep-interfering behavior. If sleep does not come quickly, the behavioral association of bed equals sleep is improved by getting out of the bed for a nonelectronic "quiet and boring" activity such as sitting in a chair to read and returning to bed only when feeling sleepy. A list of sleep hygiene practices appears in Chapter 14, "Psychosocial Interventions."

Sleep is also impaired by distracting thoughts, worries, or symptoms of many different DSM-5 conditions (Table 3–8). Addressing problems such as maltreatment, PTSD, anxiety, and mood disorders can significantly improve sleep. In some cases, insomnia worsens or perpetuates a mood disorder to such a degree that using a medication for the restoration of adequate sleep can be a way to help resolve that mood disorder more quickly.

Reasonable bedtimes may be a sticking point worth addressing. Caregivers cannot expect adolescents to fall asleep at 8:00 P.M. every night, even though that may be a reasonable expectation for younger children. For children with long-term sleep phase advancement problems, such as rarely falling asleep before 3:00 A.M., changing bedtimes too quickly does not work because it takes weeks to retrain the circadian rhythm and behavioral associations with sleep.

Obstructive sleep apnea also can have negative psychiatric effects; thus, when apnea is found in a (typically obese) child through polysomnography, a sleep apnea treatment also may improve other psychiatric symptoms. When the tonsils are large, a simple tonsillectomy or adenoidectomy may be helpful. Any more extensive surgical intervention on the palate or pharynx of a growing child should be viewed with much greater skepticism because of higher rates of complications.

TABLE 3–8. Sleep problems

Diagnostic category	Suggested screening questions
First consider	
Abuse	*"Has anything or anyone made you feel uncomfortable or unsafe?"* (for caregiver) *"Has anything happened to your child that really shouldn't have happened?"*
Bullying	*"Have other kids been teasing you or making you feel afraid?"*
Poor sleep habits	*"What is your routine before going to bed? What do you do when you cannot sleep?"*
Common diagnostic possibilities	
Generalized anxiety disorder	*"Do you feel tense, restless, or worried most of the time? Do these worries keep you awake?"*
Insomnia disorder	*"Have you had difficulty with sleep 3 or more nights a week for at least the past 3 months?"*
Major depressive disorder	*"Have you felt really down, depressed, or uninterested in things you used to enjoy for more than 2 weeks?"*
Posttraumatic stress disorder	*"Do you avoid reminders of traumatic events in your past? Do you startle easily or get frequent nightmares?"*

Continuous positive airway pressure (CPAP) systems can be effective and safe for sleep apnea treatment, but it is typically quite difficult to get a child to actually use a CPAP machine every night—far more often, these systems are purchased but not used. Notably, with severe sleep apnea, potent sedatives such as benzodiazepines at night would not be recommended.

Parents and patients often ask for a prescribed medication to help with sleep. The challenges of this strategy include limitations in effectiveness, creating psychological associations that one cannot sleep without a pill, physiological dependence or tolerance, and exposure to unwanted adverse effects. After sleep hygiene measures fail, for moderate to severe insomnia we consider a medication. The core principle should be to favor nonaddictive, safe, and low–side effect sedative options with children. The secondary principle is that if a child has insomnia plus another psychiatric disorder, selecting a medication that can address both conditions at once is preferred to using multiple medications.

Antihistamines are a reasonable first-line option because of their safety profile. Melatonin, up to 5 mg nightly, is considered generally safe, but at least theoretical concerns exist for the negative effects it may have on other hormone systems. More potent sedative options include the α-agonists (clonidine, guanfacine), which, when administered nightly, could help with sleep in addition to other conditions such as ADHD. Anxiety that continues to cause insomnia despite the use of SSRIs and CBT may benefit from hydroxyzine as a nonaddictive option or an off-label trial of a sedating antidepressant such as mirtazapine. In severe cases, a low dose of a benzodiazepine or an off-label benzodiazepine analogue (zolpidem, zaleplon) might be necessary to achieve results. For children requiring an antipsychotic to treat their psychiatric disorder, a sedating option such as quetiapine or risperidone taken at bedtime may improve the comorbid insomnia. Use of an antipsychotic solely as a sleep aid is inappropriate and unsafe (McVoy and Findling 2013).

Self-Harm and Suicidality

Suicidality and self-harm behaviors are very common among adolescents, more common than most of us realize (Table 3–9). In research surveys, 14%–24% of adolescents self-reported that they have committed an act of self-harm, and about 6%–7% stated that they have made a suicide attempt in the previous year (Lewis and Heath 2015). Thankfully, completed suicides are far more rare than the number of suicide attempts. You are more likely to get full and honest answers about suicidality and substance abuse when interviewing a young person away from his or her caregivers, so ask for privacy before you ask about self-harm.

Asking young people if they feel suicidal can be awkward until you become accustomed to asking about it. Despite the awkward feelings, these questions cannot be avoided. Be-

TABLE 3–9. Self-harm and suicidality

Diagnostic category	Suggested screening questions
First consider	
Risk acuity[a]	*"Have you ever thought about hurting yourself or taking your own life? Have you ever done something to hurt yourself or tried to kill yourself? Do you have any plans now for how you would kill yourself?"*
Current triggers[a]	*"Do you have any recent relationship problems or big disappointments?"*
Current supports[a]	*"Do you have anyone in your life who helps support you?"*
Access to lethal means[a]	*"Can you easily get a gun or enough pills that you think could kill you?"*
Common diagnostic possibilities	
Bipolar disorder	*"Has there ever been a period of a week or more when you were the opposite of depressed, with super high energy and little need for sleep?"*
Persistent depressive disorder (dysthymia)	*"Have you felt persistently sad or gloomy for more than a year?"*
Major depressive disorder	*"Have you felt really down, depressed, or uninterested in things you used to enjoy for more than 2 weeks?"*
Substance use disorder[a]	*"Have you been using drugs or alcohol?"*

[a]These questions should be asked when the patient is alone.

cause suicide is one of the three leading causes of death among the young, asking a young person about feelings of suicide is just as important as screening an adult for chest pain or shortness of breath.

If you fear that asking about suicide creates risks, allow us to put your mind at ease. Asking about suicidal thoughts, plans, and past actions not only gathers essential diagnostic information but also shows your concern. For a self-harming or suicidal young person, having an adult in her life who communicates that she cares about her is therapeutic.

When asking about suicidality, we suggest starting with broad questions, then getting specific. Asking *"Have you ever..."* risk questions before *"How about now..."* questions just flows better conversationally. If you uncover self-harming or suicidal behaviors, continuing to ask questions about previous suicidal behaviors (the strongest predictor of future behavior), current self-harm plans, and current stressors is key to being able to understand the immediacy of any risks. If you learn that the adolescent tried to avoid premature discovery of a suicide attempt, such as hiding emptied pill bottles, this would be very concerning. Easy, impulsive access to lethal means, such as a loaded firearm, is another major risk factor.

Recurrent self-harm behaviors, such as cutting, are often cited by young people themselves as a coping mechanism that they perform in part to reduce their risk of suicide. However, recurrent self-harm increases the risk for future suicidal behaviors.

The strongest predictors of a future suicide completion are a history of suicide attempts, an active mood disorder, current substance abuse, and a family history of suicidal behavior. For adolescents in particular, suicide attempts are often triggered after an acute loss or disappointment, such as breakup with a boyfriend or girlfriend or an acute family conflict. Nearly 90% of adolescent suicide deaths occur from firearms or suffocation, which includes hanging, so suicidal plans involving these strategies are the most concerning (Eaton et al. 2008). Suicide attempts by overdose are much more common but are also much less likely to be lethal.

After learning both the general and the specific details of the situation, we suggest keeping in mind a prudent layperson standard for when to consider an acute hospitalization. Child mental health specialists are not really much better than anyone else would be in assessing risks once all the details of the situation are known. The difference is that child mental health specialists excel at eliciting the details of a situation. The key is to keep asking for more information to flesh out the whole situation rather than stopping your inquiries at "they said they feel suicidal." You should consider hospitalization for any young person who appears to have a significant safety risk after you elicit the details of the situation. Psychiatric hospitalization keeps a patient physically safe for at least a short time while initiating further steps in her care.

Young people with recurrent self-harm behavior or significant suicidal thoughts should be referred for psychotherapy because this is clearly the most effective treatment available. If a family declines to use counseling with a mental health professional, you can also encourage the use of as many other social supports and supervision arrangements as possible.

Medications do not have a significant role in reducing suicide or self-harm risks on a short-term basis. However, if a child has major depressive disorder or an anxiety disorder, then long-term suicide risks can be reduced through successful treatment with SSRIs. See Chapter 15, "Psychotherapeutic Interventions," for more information about SSRI use and suicidality. For a severe depression, the greatest treatment responses occur when SSRIs are combined with psychotherapy. Frequent monitoring and making the environment safe (i.e., restricting access to dangerous medications and firearms) are advised for all suicidal young people.

Substance Abuse

The key to making any diagnosis is thinking of the possibility, which can be a challenge when it comes to adolescent substance abuse (Table 3–10). When we see fresh-faced, youthful adolescents in our offices, we can find it hard to simultaneously view them as possible substance abusers. The available statistics dictate that we do so. In the United States alone, national surveys show that past-month adolescent alcohol use rates in the United States are about 9% of 14 - to 15-year-olds and 23% of 16- to 17-year-olds, and for marijuana, about 7% of 12- to 17-year-olds report past-month use. Cocaine, hallucinogens, and inhalants are also abused by adolescents but at rates of less than 1% (Substance Abuse and Mental Health Services Administration 2014).

TABLE 3–10. Substance abuse

Diagnostic category	Suggested screening questions
First consider	
Safety[a]	*"Have you ever been in a car driven by someone who was drunk or high? Have you injured yourself while you were drunk or high? Have you blacked out or done things you regret while drunk or high?"*
Common diagnostic possibilities	
Substance use disorder[a]	*"Have people asked you to cut down on drinking or using drugs? Do you ever drink or use drugs when you are alone? Do you get strong cravings or end up using more than you wanted to?"*
Substance withdrawal	*"Do you get more moody or anxious while your alcohol or drugs are wearing off?"*
Substance tolerance	*"Has the same amount of drug or alcohol been losing its effect over time?"*
Substance/medication-induced mental disorder	*"Did you develop more mood or anxiety problems after you started using?"*
"Self-medication" role of substances	*"Are there any problems that you wanted the alcohol or drugs to resolve?"*

[a]These questions should be asked when the patient is alone.

Recognition starts with remembering to ask about substance use and ideally doing so without a parent in the room. We prefer to ask parents to leave the room for this aspect of the encounter and openly reemphasize applicable confidentiality rules during the separation process. Generally, everyone will understand the concept of maintaining confidentiality unless a major safety risk exists, such as having blackouts or driving while intoxicated. This same one-on-one time can be used to discuss other sensitive topics such as self-harm and suicidality.

A widely recommended screening tool for adolescents is the CRAFFT (Figure 3–1), which the American Academy of Pediatrics recommends using during adolescent health maintenance appointments (Yuma-Guerrero et al. 2012). If two or more question answers are positive, there is a high chance of a substance use disorder being present (Knight et al. 2002).

Urine drug testing may help to evaluate the cause of an acute intoxication or may be used for tracking care within a specialized substance abuse treatment program. However, we do not otherwise recommend urine drug testing as a part of routine care because it can unnecessarily diminish the therapeutic alliance.

In the past, the emphasis was on needing to determine whether a patient's substance use represented abuse or dependence. Because this differentiation was often unclear and carried both stigma and legal ramifications, these separate dependence and abuse diagnoses were merged into a single substance use disorder diagnosis in DSM-5. The hallmarks of a substance use disorder include loss of control over one's use, social impairments, use in risky situations or despite negative consequences, and physiological changes of tolerance or withdrawal. In other words, not all adolescents who use substances have a disorder.

You should be alert to symptoms caused by substance abuse that look like another psychiatric illness. Sedative drugs (hypnotics, anxiolytics, and alcohol) can cause depression during intoxication but anxiety during withdrawal. Stimulating drugs (amphetamines, cocaine) can cause psychosis and anxiety during intoxication but depression during withdrawal. Both drug classes cause sexual and sleep disturbances. Psychotic symptoms may occur from anticholinergics, cardiovascular drugs, steroids, stimulants, and depressants. Marijuana can cause depressed mood and anxiety, even though adolescents claim that it treats their depression or anxiety. In an adolescent vulnerable to psychosis, marijuana can trigger persisting psychotic symptoms (van Nierop and Janssens 2013).

When substance-created psychiatric symptoms are possible, we motivate the adolescent to do a self-test of not using for a specific period of time (e.g., at least 2 weeks) to see what happens. Most substance-induced mental disorders will im-

Begin: "I'm going to ask you a few questions that I ask all my patients. Please be honest. I will keep your answers confidential."

Part A

During the PAST 12 MONTHS, did you:

	No	Yes
1. Drink any <u>alcohol</u> (more than a few sips)? (Do not count a few sips of alcohol taken during family or religious events)	☐	☐
2. Smoke any <u>marijuana or hashish?</u>	☐	☐
3. Use <u>anything else</u> to get high? ("anything else" includes illegal drugs, synthetic marijuana, over-the-counter and prescription drugs, or things that people sniff or "huff")	☐	☐

FIGURE 3–1. The CRAFFT Screening Interview.

Source. © John R. Knight, MD, Boston Children's Hospital, 2015. All rights reserved. Reproduced with permission. For more information, contact ceasar@childrens.harvard.edu.

For clinic use only: Did the patient answer "yes" to any questions in Part A?

No ☐ → Ask CAR question only, then stop

Yes ☐ → Ask all 6 CRAFFT questions

Part B

	No	Yes
1. Have you ever ridden in a **CAR** driven by someone (including yourself) who was "high" or had been using alcohol or drugs?	☐	☐
2. Do you ever use alcohol or drugs to **RELAX**, feel better about yourself, or fit in?	☐	☐
3. Do you ever use alcohol or drugs while you are by yourself, or **ALONE**?	☐	☐
4. Do you ever **FORGET** things you did while using alcohol or drugs?	☐	☐
5. Do your **FAMILY** or **FRIENDS** ever tell you that you should cut down on your drinking or drug use?	☐	☐
6. Have you ever gotten into **TROUBLE** while you were using alcohol or drugs?	☐	☐

*Two or more **YES** answers on the CRAFFT suggest a serious problem and need for further assessment.

FIGURE 3–1. The CRAFFT Screening Interview. *(continued)*

prove after a few weeks of abstinence. For adolescents who say "I can stop whenever I want to," we would follow this statement by empowering them to do just that for the reasons that make the most sense to them. This does two things: 1) it determines whether their symptoms really are substance induced, and 2) if they cannot go more than 2 weeks without using, then it highlights their lack control over their use.

Care of a substance use disorder is based on educating adolescents about the negative outcomes from use, helping them learn their triggers and motivating reasons to use, building motivation for change, and shaping family involvement in resolving the problem. Motivational interviewing, CBT, family therapy, supervised peer groups, mindfulness training, identifying triggers (to avoid future cue-based use), changing peer groups, and arranging for rewards for evidence of sobriety are all specific outpatient care options.

Disturbed Eating

Eating disorders such as anorexia and bulimia can present a diagnostic challenge in that young people who have become significantly ill with an eating disorder generally try to hide their symptoms, even when asked directly by a trusted person (Table 3–11). With low-weight anorexia nervosa particular, withholding information or even lying to practitioners often happens in the service of maintaining disordered eating. Therapists sometimes refer to these lies as the eating disorder, rather than the patient herself, doing the talking. Because of this inconsistency, collateral informants (i.e., parents and other caregivers) are typically very helpful for understanding the extent of symptoms and behaviors. An investigative approach helps. When you learn that a young person who denies self-induced vomiting goes to the bathroom immediately after most of her meals, you should explore the possibility of disturbed eating and body image. Remember that young people with eating disorders often show rigid thinking and perfectionism.

Postpartum Maternal Mental Health

Maternal peripartum depression is common, even more so in developing countries (about 1 in 5) than in developed countries (about 1 in 10) (Paschetta et al. 2014). The risk that the

TABLE 3–11. Disturbed eating

Diagnostic category	Suggested screening questions
First consider	
Medically induced weight loss	*"Have you had recurring diarrhea?"* (inflammatory bowel disease) *Have you been losing weight despite wanting to maintain?"* (endocrine disorder/malignancy)
Self-harm[a]	*"Have you been thinking about hurting yourself? Have you ever hurt yourself or attempted suicide?"*
Common diagnostic possibilities	
Anorexia nervosa	*"Do you worry about losing control when you eat? Do you prefer to eat alone?"* (on growth curve: an unexpected loss of weight or failure to gain appropriately)
Bulimia nervosa	*"Have you had recurring times when you overeat and then feel the need to compensate afterward? Do you use laxatives or vomit after meals?"*
Major depressive disorder	*"Have you felt really down, depressed, or uninterested in things you used to enjoy for more than 2 weeks?"*
Substance use disorder[a]	*"Have you been using drugs or alcohol?"*

[a]These questions should be asked when the patient is alone.

mother of a newborn will experience depression increases with stressors such as poverty, lack of partner support, unwanted pregnancy, and domestic violence. When a woman has depressive symptoms during her pregnancy, the chances that she will develop postpartum depression increase, so we counsel increased vigilance for these parents.

Postdelivery obstetric care for mothers and the first year of health maintenance care for children ideally include some form of screening for maternal depressive and anxiety problems (Table 3–12). You can accomplish this by conversationally asking the mother about her psychological well-being (which helps to communicate its importance) and can supplement this approach with a brief rating scale screen (such as the Patient Health Questionnaire 9-item or Generalized Anxiety Disorder 7-item scale) in routine office care. Fatigue and poor sleep, which are often associated with parenthood itself, need to be recognized as potential signs of an episode of major depressive disorder.

Good parental mental health is important for children. When parents struggle, there can be negative effects on the child's physical state (poor health, poor weight gain), cognitive status (delayed acquisition of milestones, impaired attention), social development (ODD, conduct problems), behavior (more crying, irritability, and temperament challenges), and emotional development (depression, anxiety) (Satyanarayana et al. 2011). In rare instances, a parental mental health condition can become so severe, such as developing psychosis, that a parent will actually harm her child.

Treating parental mental health problems during a child's early development phase has been found to have positive effects on child mental health. When a parent or other caregiver with mental illness receives care, this also greatly increases the chance that the child will develop an easygoing temperament, which will pay dividends in the household for years (Hanington et al. 2010).

Treating a parent or caregiver begins with addressing life stressors ranging from mild (keeping up with laundry or cleaning) to severe (loss of employment, poor relationship with partner). Rallying a parent's personal care system to support her and take her distress seriously may be sufficient to produce positive change. Psychotherapy is indicated for any situations in which major depression, GAD, or another significant disorder has set in.

The decision to use psychiatric medications postpartum is similar to what one would choose at any other time for mental health treatment. The degree of psychiatric medication transmission through breast milk is typically too low to generate any effects on a breast-feeding child, with the notable exception of lithium (Davanzo et al. 2011). Moderate to severe depression generally responds most quickly to a combination of SSRIs and psychotherapy, so this should be the usual approach (Lanza di Scalea and Wisner 2009).

TABLE 3–12. Postpartum maternal mental health

Diagnostic category	Suggested screening questions
First consider	
Suicidality	*"Have you been having thoughts about hurting yourself?"*
Psychosis	*"Have you been hearing voices or feeling worried that your mind is playing tricks on you?"*
Child safety	*"Have you felt worried that you might intentionally hurt your child?"*
Common diagnostic possibilities	
Anxiety disorder	*"Do you feel tense or worried most of the time? Do worries affect your sleep?"*
Major depressive disorder	*"Have you felt really down, depressed, or uninterested in things you used to enjoy for more than 2 weeks?"*

Medication choices during pregnancy itself have to be weighed a bit more carefully against the potential effects a specific medication may have on a developing fetus. The traditional advice was to avoid lithium because of the risk of Ebstein's anomaly, but recent research (Pearlstein 2013) identifies those congenital defects of the tricuspid valve as more rare than previously believed. Lithium may be prescribed, with caution and counseling, during pregnancy. We do, however, advise against the use of valproate, a known teratogen whose maternal use is associated with neurodevelopmental disorders in children. The rare, but well-reported, risk of low birth weight or pulmonary hypertension of the newborn from SSRI use during pregnancy means that SSRIs should be reserved for more severe cases of depression and anxiety (Pearlstein 2013).

Any time a parent develops psychosis or suicidality, a hospital admission level of care should be considered.

Chapter 4

The 15-Minute Pediatric Diagnostic Interview

Even the most seasoned and skilled practitioner would like to have at least 30 minutes to perform a diagnostic mental health interview. Determining the character traits, cognitive ability, and emotional health of another person, especially a child or an adolescent, is difficult. So why even discuss a 15-minute diagnostic interview?

Short diagnostic mental health interviews are not ideal, but the reality is that they are performed with young people every day. Primary care and emergency department practitioners are routinely expected to perform very quick interviews. Pediatric primary care practitioners can be expected to evaluate as many as 30 different children per day, which leaves only about 15 minutes to spend with each patient. Emergency department practitioners are pressured to rapidly assess mental health concerns, particularly during evening hours when emergency environments are most stressed.

The time available for performing a mental health evaluation is further constrained when a patient or family is focused on physical health concerns instead. By the time your assessment identifies a psychiatric issue—the anxiety that precedes vague abdominal pain or the dsyphoria that is experienced as a headache—you may have only a few minutes remaining in an appointment to conduct a full mental health diagnostic assessment. Patients also may have the "Oh, by the way..." moments, when major mental health questions are broached seemingly as a practitioner places his hand on the door to leave the examination room.

Practitioners frequently find their available time restricted in one way or another, so it helps to think about how to best use even a small amount of time to advance the care of children and adolescents with mental distress.

The following five steps are one way to efficiently perform a focused mental health diagnostic assessment with a child or an adolescent. Even under time constraints, you can build a therapeutic alliance and develop an initial treatment plan by following these five steps.

1. Prescreen mental health concerns with a validated tool.
2. Identify the leading concerns.
3. Identify and address safety issues.
4. Diagnose a probable or unspecified disorder.
5. Recommend a next step.

Step 1: Prescreen Mental Health Concerns With a Validated Tool

We recommend the use of pre-interview assessment tools as a standard part of the workup for well-child visits but especially when the chief complaint is a mental or behavioral health problem. Preassessment screening tools engage a patient and his caregivers in the treatment, normalize conversations about mental distress, and assist you in identifying the chief complaint. Several brief screening instruments for a wide variety of mental health concerns are available. One example is the DSM-5 (American Psychiatric Association 2013) Level 1 Cross-Cutting Symptom Measure, which lists selected symptoms of major DSM-5 disorders in a brief format. Versions exist for caregivers of children and adolescents between ages 6 and 17 and for patients between ages 11 and 17. These measures are free and can be reproduced for clinical use and are referenced further in Chapter 10, "Selected DSM-5 Assessment Measures." We also recommend considering use of the Pediatric Symptom Checklist or the Strengths and Difficulties Questionnaire, two other brief but broad-based assessment measures that have the additional benefit of score validation for children in primary care medical settings.

Whatever screening tool you select for your practice setting, you should familiarize yourself with its scoring system. Most screening tools are designed to have high sensitivity, meaning that they aim to identify anyone who may have a particular diagnosis, but lower specificity, meaning that they will identify some persons for additional concern who ultimately will not have the diagnosis for which you are screening. Positive results in certain categories may suggest follow-up measures to use, such as a high inattention score on the DSM-5

Level 1 assessment being followed up with the DSM-5 Level 2 Inattention rating scale. Using follow-up measures can increase the efficiency of a clinic and, if patients are followed up over time, can be a good introduction to using validated scales to measure treatment response, relapse, and recovery. At the very least, the results of screening measures also can be used as conversation starters: *"I see that you indicated a few concerns in the questionnaire; can you tell me more about that?"*

Although the use of brief, broad screening measures is likely best for a fast-paced care facility, if time and the practice plan allow, a more detailed symptom checklist should be considered instead. Tools such as the Behavior Assessment System for Children (Reynolds and Kamphaus 1998) and the Child Behavior Checklist (Achenbach 1991, 1992) take significantly more time for caregivers to complete and for office staff to score and interpret, but once completed, they result in reliable, broad-based pictures of a young person's difficulties.

If you fail to recognize the presence of a mental health concern in advance, you can still choose to pause the evaluation process when such concerns arise and ask for the symptom screening information to be completed before continuing. For instance, you may say, *"Given the concerns you just raised, could you take a few moments to complete this information, and I'll be back to discuss this more with you?"* Taking this approach could allow you to proceed with seeing your next scheduled patient during that time and even have the assessment tool scored by an assistant while staying on schedule.

When you have identified a specific mental health concern, a condition- or symptom-focused rating scale could be used instead to provide better diagnostic information. Examples of focused DSM-5 scales include the Level 2 Cross-Cutting Symptom Measures for parents or children to characterize symptom categories such as anger, anxiety, depression, inattention, irritability, mania, sleep disturbance, somatic symptoms, and substance use; these scales are discussed in Chapter 10 in brief but are also available online (www.psychiatry.org/practice/dsm/dsm5/online-assessment-measures#Level2). Other symptom-focused scales have been validated and normed with diagnostic score cutoffs in children and are discussed in Chapter 11, "Rating Scales and Alternative Diagnostic Systems." Positive results on these instruments more strongly suggest that a particular diagnosis is present, but the use of a diagnostic instrument ultimately relies on the prudent judgment of a practitioner.

Even the best rating scales and symptom checklists are inherently imperfect, so it is important to understand their limitations. Questions may be misunderstood, may miss key symptoms, may be influenced by a young person's or caregiver's tendency to overreport or underreport symptoms, or may be intentionally answered untruthfully. This is why all surveys and questionnaires must be followed up with a personalized diagnostic interview to yield a more complete and reliable picture. For instance, if we see an adolescent who denied having depression symptoms on his rating scale yet appears withdrawn, speaks in a low monotone, and describes feeling hopeless, then depression must be considered, regardless of the scores on a symptom checklist.

Step 2: Identify the Leading Concerns

Once a pertinent rating scale has been completed and scored, the next step in a brief interview is to identify the young person's and caregiver's leading concern for further investigation. Identifying the leading concern can be as simple as asking specifically, *"What are you most concerned about today?"*

An unlimited list of concerns or complaints is too challenging to manage within a brief investigation, even if the concerns ultimately relate to the same diagnosis, as is often the case with depression. For instance, a family may describe sleep problems, poor academic performance, self-harm behavior, irritability, and conflict with a sibling as separate concerns. If you identify one of these areas, such as self-harm, as the chief concern for that day, with the understanding that remaining concerns such as sibling conflict may need to be addressed at another appointment, then a 15-minute interview can be more fruitful.

Your own careful judgment is the key. For example, if a patient and his caregivers are most concerned about sleep disturbances but your screening tools or examination alert you to a safety issue, you must explain to the family that sleep disturbances are important, but the patient's safety is the leading concern at present.

Having the patient and his caregivers each identify a leading concern builds your therapeutic alliance and increases investment in your assessment and treatment. When a patient and his caregivers believe that you truly understand the leading concern, they are more likely to engage in treatment and follow the next steps you recommend.

Step 3: Identify and Address Safety Issues

Any mental health evaluation, no matter how brief, includes an assessment of safety. If you identify safety concerns, then the near-term care plan needs to account for how to reduce or eliminate that risk.

- If you suspect that self-harm or suicidal behaviors may occur, as when evaluating for depression, ask: "*Do you ever think about hurting yourself? Have you ever deliberately hurt yourself?*"
- If it is possible that abuse or neglect may be related to the reported symptoms, ask: "*Has anything made you feel uncomfortable or unsafe? Has anyone ever tried to hurt you?*"
- If it is possible that the child poses a risk to another person, ask: "*Have you ever hurt someone else on purpose? Do you have any plans to do that now?*"

Step 4: Diagnose a Probable or Unspecified Disorder

By inquiring about the circumstances and details surrounding a patient's (and his caregiver's) chief concern and reviewing the results of assessment tools, a practitioner can usually arrive at a probable diagnosis in 15 minutes. Confirmation of all but the most obvious diagnoses will take more assessment time or a future appointment to clarify. For instance, you might determine in just 15 minutes that a child has significant developmental impairments, leading to a diagnosis of unspecified neurodevelopmental disorder. Then, during his next appointment you would make more detailed inquiries to refine the diagnosis further, changing that diagnosis to something more specific such as a language disorder or an autism spectrum disorder.

In Chapter 3, "Common Clinical Concerns," we outline the more likely diagnoses to consider and some specific screening questions you can use when confronted with common pediatric concerns.

Rapid assessments proceed more fruitfully with awareness of the key aspects of common clinical conditions. This is no different from the rest of medicine, in which shorthand understandings of disorders are used to guide clinical suspicion. When an adult reports chest pain radiating down his left arm, we suspect a heart attack. When a febrile infant pulls at his ears and acts grumpy, we suspect an ear infection. In a similar way, we can learn to recognize basic patterns of mental health. When a child experiences several weeks of a persistently low mood and loses interest in the activities and friends he usually enjoys, we suspect major depressive disorder. To help inform your clinical suspicion, Table 4–1 contains a list of common psychiatric conditions and shorthand descriptions. Additional information is available in later chapters.

Remember that these are descriptions of behaviors and symptoms. In isolation, these behaviors are not a diagnosis. In the DSM-5 diagnostic system, for any constellation of behaviors and symptoms to qualify as a psychiatric diagnosis, they must meet two conditions:

1. They cause a significant functional impairment.
2. They are not better explained by another etiology.

The second rule is very important. A child can be inattentive for any number of reasons without having attention-deficit/hyperactivity disorder, and an adolescent can be sad for many reasons without experiencing a major depressive episode. If these kinds of behaviors and symptoms do not significantly impair function or can be better explained by another etiology, a formal mental health diagnosis should not be made. You can (and should) plan to follow up with the child or adolescent to see how these symptoms develop over time.

Under DSM-IV (American Psychiatric Association 1994), a disorder that did not meet full diagnostic criteria but still met the two conditions described earlier could be labeled as a *not otherwise specified* (NOS) condition. DSM-IV's NOS diagnosis allowed a clinician to initiate treatment for a patient whose presentation was not consistent with a more specific diagnosis. The heterogeneity of this category discouraged research, frustrated epidemiology, and diminished the clinical utility of diagnoses (Fairburn and Bohn 2005). These diagnos-

TABLE 4–1. Shorthand descriptions of common DSM-5 diagnoses in children

Attention-deficit/ hyperactivity disorder	Developmentally inappropriate and persistent difficulty with inattention and/or hyperactivity with symptoms present in multiple settings
Anorexia nervosa	Restrictive eating and food avoidance, often with an accompanying desire to avoid obesity, which persists despite negative consequences
Autism spectrum disorder	A developmentally inappropriate and persistent pattern of predominant impairments in social relatedness and restricted interests and behaviors
Bipolar disorder	Discrete episode of elevated mood for multiple days with rapid thoughts, decreased need for sleep, persisting high energy, and unusual risk taking
Bulimia nervosa	More than 3 months of recurring episodes of binge eating followed by an intense desire to compensate afterward (e.g., by purging or using laxatives)
Conduct disorder	Repetitive significant violations of social rules and the rights of others over the course of a year
Encopresis	Inappropriate stool leakage with psychological adaptations, usually facilitated by chronic constipation
Generalized anxiety disorder	More than 6 months of persisting but diffuse, changing worries for more days than not that cause symptoms such as tension, fatigue, irritability, and poor concentration
Major depressive disorder	More than 2 weeks of low (or irritable) mood coupled with new neurovegetative symptoms (e.g., loss of concentration, low energy, altered sleep or appetite)

TABLE 4–1. Shorthand descriptions of common DSM-5 diagnoses in children *(continued)*

Obsessive-compulsive disorder	Time-consuming internal repetition of unwanted thoughts and/or a persistent focus on repeating specific types of behaviors or mental acts (e.g., cleaning, counting)
Oppositional defiant disorder	Developmentally inappropriate opposition to and defiance of adult rules and requests for more than 6 months
Panic attack	Sudden worry or fear accompanied by body symptoms such as a racing heart rate and physiological arousal (panic disorder considered if recurring attacks are feared and are affecting function)
Phobia (social or specific)	Excessive fear of an object or a situation that causes a dysfunctional degree of avoidance and distress for >6 months
Posttraumatic stress disorder	A traumatic experience has led to avoidance of trauma reminders, hypervigilance to future threats, and unwanted reexperiencing (including nightmares) for >1 month

Source. American Psychiatric Association 2013.

tic labels were frequently used in children and adolescents. For example, in a recent national survey of outpatient visits to physicians in the United States, 35% of all visits to physicians for mental health problems resulted in an NOS diagnosis for children and adolescents, and the number of NOS visits grew proportionally over the decade analyzed by the researchers (Safer et al. 2015). NOS diagnoses tend, over time, to be neither reliable nor valid, so they are a poor foundation for an ongoing treatment plan.

In an effort to reverse this trend, DSM-5 removed the NOS option in favor of *other specified* and *unspecified* disorders. The unspecified and other specified criteria found in each chapter of DSM-5 provide more details than the comparable NOS sections in DSM-IV. In general, practitioners are advised to consider an *unspecified* diagnosis when a young person experiences symptoms characteristic of a mental disorder that cause clinically significant distress but do not meet the full criteria for a named diagnosis. If a practitioner wishes to communicate the specific reason that symptoms in a child or an adolescent do not meet criteria, the practitioner is encouraged to use the *other specified* diagnosis. In a 15-minute diagnostic interview, practitioners may be more likely to arrive at unspecified diagnostic labels rather than full diagnoses, but this should be a reminder of the need for additional diagnostic clarification later. Children and adolescents deserve the most accurate diagnosis possible.

Step 5: Recommend a Next Step

Treat versus refer decisions end up being based on patient factors, such as diagnosis and severity, along with the fit between a patient's treatment needs and your abilities and availabilities as a practitioner and the type of services available in your local community.

Therapist Referral

For nearly every moderate or severe mental health problem, referring a child or an adolescent to a skilled mental health therapist is essential. Explaining why you think seeing a therapist will be helpful may increase motivation for patients and caregivers to follow through on your referral. If caregivers have reservations about working with a mental health practitioner, it helps to address those concerns during the referral and to normalize the referral by saying something like "*Just as I would refer you to a specialist to examine your eyes if I thought you needed glasses, I recommend that you see a mental health specialist for the concerns we have identified together.*"

Family- and Self-Help-Delivered Interventions

For low-severity problems, it may be appropriate to provide coaching on behavior or life management changes a patient and his caregivers can make at home. Providing guidance on how to improve sleep hygiene, to manage a problem behavior, or to support a young person through a life adjustment is an everyday occurrence for most primary care practitioners, and we provide some guidance in Chapter 14, "Psychosocial Interventions." Handout instructions, books, videos, or Web sites so that the family can obtain additional guidance after the appointment also may be of assistance.

Educational Assessment

For children struggling in school for whom a learning disability is a consideration, we advocate for educational testing. The route for doing this may hinge on motivating the parent to make a written request for a learning disability assessment at the child's school, which is required in some settings, including the United States.

Early Intervention Services Referral

For very young children with developmental concerns, refer the child to a local early intervention program. In the United States, this involves the federally sponsored Zero to Three program (http://zerotothree.org) or a school district–sponsored program for children ages 4–5 years.

Safety Plan

For a significant suicide, homicide, or other behavior-related safety risk, an immediate safety plan or hospitalization should be explored with the local mental health crisis system. For milder risks such as depression without active suicidal thoughts or plans, appropriate parental supervision and monitoring would be enough to detect any worsening risks.

Medications

It is usually inappropriate to recommend a new long-term psychotropic medication after only a 15-minute assessment. The exception might be a short-term trial of an over-the-counter medication with low medical side-effect risks, such as melatonin to help with insomnia. However, after a second appointment or any evaluation of a longer duration when the diagnosis becomes more certain, a prescription may be appropriate. Whenever you suspect more severe health disorders, such as bipolar disorder or schizophrenia, you should refer a patient and his caregivers immediately to a specialty mental health practitioner.

Follow-Up Appointment

If you identify a mental health problem, a follow-up appointment should be recommended. This can serve several purposes:

- Provide enough time to better complete the diagnostic process
- Communicate your ongoing therapeutic connection and support around the problem
- Track the response to any initial intervention so that the treatment plan can be adjusted
- Identify any problems with the referral plan, creating an opportunity for resolution

Chapter 5

The 30-Minute Pediatric Diagnostic Interview

Every interview with a young person with mental distress will be unique. Sometimes you will need to calm a screaming child or warm up a reluctant adolescent before you can ask any diagnostic questions. In moments like those, it sometimes feels like you are wasting time. You have other people to see and other tasks to attend to. However, good interviewers learn to receive these moments as part of the interview itself. They watch and listen to the child or adolescent for clues about whether the distress is internal or external and what events bring her into and out of engagement with a practitioner.

Every young person is also unique, so we begin an initial encounter by getting to know the child or adolescent we are seeing. We use different strategies depending on the child's age and developmental status, the location in which we are meeting, our familiarity with the patient, the patient's sense of humor, and many other variables. Before introducing ourselves to a patient, we like to know how long she has been waiting and with whom. A child who has sat calmly for 15 minutes in a waiting room will likely have different needs from the same child who has been waiting hours to see you in the emergency department. When we meet a patient, we prefer to open the conversation with a topic in which the child or adolescent is already engaged. If a young child brings a stuffed animal to an appointment or wears a colorful shirt, we ask about it. If an adolescent brings a book or is listening to music, we ask her to describe the book or song. The point is not to make an aesthetic judgment about the stuffed animals, clothes, books, and music with which a young person presents but to understand how she thinks.

Asking about something that the patient is consciously (or unconsciously) presenting to you also builds the therapeutic alliance. Imagine if you walked into a medical encounter and your physician began asking you about her interests but waved off any attempts to discuss your own. You, like most of us, would feel ignored and would likely be reluctant to engage in treatment with the physician. Now imagine if you visited another physician and she knew your name, said it correctly, and then asked how you came by your name. You would likely be more engaged with this second physician and her treatment. You can (and should) extend the same engaging courtesy to the children and adolescents you meet as patients.

We favor beginning every interview by introducing yourself, asking the young person her name, assessing her expectations for the encounter, clarifying any misperceptions, and giving a sense of how long the encounter will last. Caregivers, rather than young people themselves, set up most evaluations, so verbally acknowledging this right away ("*So, your mom wanted you to see me….*") shows a young person that you can see things through her eyes.

When the encounter is limited to 30 minutes, we believe that you can successfully develop a therapeutic alliance and perform a diagnostic interview. Before we explain how, we need to offer a few caveats.

- Any psychiatric examination that obtains all the information from a single source is incomplete. This is especially true when interviewing a child or an adolescent. You should disclose to the person you are interviewing that you will be speaking to some of her adult caregivers about her health and what you will be discussing. See Chapter 3, "Common Clinical Concerns," and Chapter 10, "Selected DSM-5 Assessment Measures," for tools to use in interviewing adult caregivers.
- A successful psychiatric examination ultimately provides access to the internal world of a person. The thoughts, impulses, and desires of a young person can be engaged in many ways. In what follows, we offer an interview that is best suited for a young person who can tolerate direct questions. When interviewing a child or an adolescent who cannot do so because of age, impairment, or disinterest, we recommend focusing on the most essential portion of the examination and spending the remainder of your time developing a therapeutic alliance.
- A skilled psychiatric examination always includes an account of the relationships that constitute a person's exis-

tence. This is especially true with children and adolescents, whose dependence on other people is more apparent than it is for the average adult. During every interview with a young person, we always ask questions such as *"Who do you live with?" "How do you spend your days?" "Who cares for you?"* and *"Who can you trust?"* These kinds of questions naturally lead into other critical questions about the caregivers in a young person's life.

With these caveats in mind, we offer the following as a guideline for a diagnostic interview that uses DSM-5 (American Psychiatric Association 2013) criteria. The interview does not include prompts for DSM-5 categories that are uncommon in childhood and adolescence—namely, the neurocognitive, gambling, paraphilia, personality, and sexual dysfunction disorders. (We do, however, provide guidance for assessing personality traits in Chapter 10.) We have taught a version of this interview to students, residents, fellows, and faculty. Until you develop the habits of an experienced practitioner, it helps to practice a structured interview. This helps in becoming comfortable asking about intimate concerns, remembering to screen all patients for the major categories of mental illness, and developing good interview habits.

Of course, a structured interview has a downside. We have sometimes witnessed practitioners read one question after another, without stopping for the usual pauses that signify human speech or even looking at the patient. In *The Pocket Guide to the DSM-5™ Diagnostic Exam* (Nussbaum 2013), we called these kinds of interviewers psychiatric robots who ask things like *"I hear you are suicidal, but can you spell* world *backward?"*—questions that show more fidelity to an outlined interview than attention to the specific person before you. These kinds of interviewers speak so stiffly and stay so determinedly on script that when witnessing them, you wonder which of their joints need to be oiled first. Trust us, we both have performed the psychiatric robot interview ourselves at some point during our careers. We wrote this guide in part so that you can learn from our mistakes.

What we found (and still find) challenging is providing the right amount of structure for the interview. An excitable person will need to be calmed, a sad person must be encouraged, and sometimes the same person will need both in the same interview. Fortunately, you always have the best possible guide: the person before you. Follow her lead. Observe her body language. If she appears disinterested, it is time to alter your approach.

As you use this diagnostic interview, strike a balance between becoming a psychiatric robot and practicing a formal version until it becomes a habit. The 30-minute diagnostic interview will seem forced at first, but gradually it provides the infrastructure for a conversational interview.

No matter how distracted or upset the patient, good interviewers always give a person a few minutes to speak her own mind. Then, they summarize and clarify the patient's concerns and organize the examination as necessary, modulating the structure and language of the interview to fit the needs of the patient. They ask clear and succinct questions. If the patient is vague, they seek precision. If she remains vague, they explore why. They do not ask permission to change the subject but use transition statements, such as "*I think I understand this, but how about that?*" Developing a supply of stock questions is helpful, which is why we advise using this structured interview until it becomes a habit. Then you can use these questions to develop a conversational style for an interview in which a patient tells her story, you form an alliance with her, you gain insight into her thought process, and you gather the clinical data needed to make an accurate diagnosis. When you do so, you reduce the patient's alienation by making the strange more familiar.

Outline of the 30-Minute Pediatric Diagnostic Interview

The interview outline in this section includes headings that indicate the time allotted for each portion of the interview (boldface type), instructions to the interviewer (roman type), and questions for the interviewer to ask (italic type).

Minute 1

Introduce yourself to the patient. Ask how she would like to be addressed. Set expectations for how long you will meet and what you will accomplish. Describe applicable limits of confidentiality with an adolescent, such as "*What we talk about will remain confidential except if there is a risk for your safety—then we would talk together with your parent about how to best keep you safe."* Then ask, *"Why are you here today?"*

Minutes 2–4

Listen

A patient's uninterrupted speech indicates much of her mental status, guides your history taking, and builds the alliance. As she speaks, listen to the content and form of her statements. What is she saying or not saying? How is she saying it? How do her statements match her appearance? Although you may be tempted to interrupt or begin asking questions, with experience, you will find that allowing the person to talk initially without interruptions gives you more information about her than the answers to your questions will. When you do speak next, try to have your question be both responsive and open ended, along the lines of *"You said ____; can you tell me more about that?"* Depending on the nature of the illness, some people will be unable to fill this time; their inability to do so also provides valuable information about their mental status and distress. When the person does not speak spontaneously, you may have to use prompts and proceed to the history of the current illness.

Minutes 5–12

History of Current Illness

Your questions should follow the DSM-5 criteria, as described in Chapter 6, "DSM-5 Pediatric Diagnostic Interview." Additionally, you should focus on what has changed recently—the "why now?" of the presentation. As you do, seek understanding of precipitating events: When did the patient's current distress begin? When was the last time she felt emotionally well? Can she identify any precipitating, perpetuating, or extenuating events? How have her thoughts and behaviors affected her psychosocial functioning? How does the patient view her current level of functioning, and how is it different from what it was days, weeks, or months ago?

Psychiatric History

"When did you first notice symptoms? When did you first seek treatment? Did you ever experience a full recovery? Have you ever

been hospitalized? How many times? What was the reason for those hospitalizations, and how long were you hospitalized? Do you receive outpatient mental health treatment? Do you take medications for a mental illness? Which medicines have helped the most? Did you have any adverse effects from any medications? What was the reason for stopping prior medications? How long were you taking each medication, and how often did you take it? Do you know the name, strength, and number of doses per day of medicines you are currently taking?"

Safety

Students and trainees may feel uncomfortable asking these questions and may worry that they will upset patients or even give them ideas about ways to hurt themselves or others. These fears are largely unfounded, and with practice you will find that these questions become much easier to ask. It is important to remember that one of the biggest predictors of future behavior is past behavior, so asking about prior episodes of violence to self and others is required for an overall risk assessment. *"Do you frequently think about hurting yourself? Have you ever hurt yourself, such as cutting or hitting? Have you ever attempted to kill yourself? How many attempts have you made? What did you do? What medical or psychiatric treatment did you receive after these attempts? Do you often become so upset that you make threats to hurt other people, animals, or property? Have you ever hurt people or animals, destroyed property, tricked other people, or stolen things?"*

Minutes 13–17

Review of Systems

The psychiatric review of systems is an overview of common psychiatric symptoms that you may not have elicited in the history of the current illness. If a person answers affirmatively to these questions, you should explore further with the DSM-5 criteria, as modeled in Chapter 6.

Mood. *"Have you been feeling sad, blue, down, depressed, or irritable? If so, does feeling this way make it hard to do things, to concentrate, or to sleep? Are you angry most of the time? Has there been a time when for many days straight your mood was super happy, you were more self-confident, and you had much more energy than usual? If so, can you describe what happened?"* (See

"Depressive Disorders" or "Bipolar and Related Disorders" in Chapter 6.)

Psychosis. *"Have you seen visions or other things that other people did not see? Have you heard noises, sounds, or voices that other people did not hear? Do you ever feel like people are following you or trying to hurt you in some way? Have you ever felt that you had special powers or found special messages from the radio or TV seemingly meant just for you?"* (See "Schizophrenia Spectrum and Other Psychotic Disorders" in Chapter 6.)

Anxiety. *"Would you say that you worry a lot or more than other kids your age? Do people say that you worry too much or are too shy? Do you feel afraid when you're alone or away from your family? Do you get scared about going to school? Is it hard for you to control or stop your worrying? Are there specific things, places, or situations that make you feel very anxious or fearful? Have you ever felt suddenly frightened, nervous, or anxious for no reason at all? If so, can you tell me about that?"* (See "Anxiety Disorders" in Chapter 6.)

Obsessions and compulsions. *"Do you ever get unwanted thoughts or pictures stuck in your mind and repeating that you cannot get rid of? Is there anything you feel you have to check, clean, or organize over and over again in order to feel OK?"* (See "Obsessive-Compulsive and Related Disorders" in Chapter 6.)

Trauma. *"What is the worst thing that has ever happened to you? Has someone ever touched you in a way you did not want? Have you ever felt that your life was in danger or thought that you were going to be seriously injured? Do you have unhappy memories that make it hard to sleep or to feel OK now?"* (See "Trauma- and Stressor-Related Disorders" in Chapter 6.)

Dissociation. *"Do people say that you daydream a lot or look spaced out? Do you lose track of time and feel unsure of what you did during that time? Do you ever feel as if you are standing outside your body or watching yourself?"* (See "Dissociative Disorders" in Chapter 6.)

Eating and feeding. *"Do you avoid particular foods so much that it affects your health or weight? Do you worry about losing control over how much you eat?"* (See "Feeding and Eating Disorders" in Chapter 6.)

Elimination. *"Have you had any problem with passing urine or feces onto your clothing or bed?"* (See "Elimination Disorders" in Chapter 6.)

The 30-Minute Pediatric Diagnostic Interview **77**

Somatic concerns. *"Do you worry about your health more than other kids do? Do you often miss school because you do not feel well? Do you get sick with aches and pains more often than most young people do?"* (See "Somatic Symptom and Related Disorders" in Chapter 6.)

Sleeping. *"Do you struggle to fall asleep, or do you wake up a lot at night? Do you often feel sleepy during the day? Has anyone said that you stop breathing or gasp for air while sleeping?"* (See "Sleep-Wake Disorders" in Chapter 6.)

Substances and other addictions. *"In the past year, have you drunk alcohol, smoked marijuana, or used anything else to get high? Have you ever ridden in a car with someone who was high or drinking alcohol? Do you ever use alcohol or drugs when you are alone? Do you ever use alcohol or drugs to relax?"* (Knight et al. 2002). (See "Substance-Related and Addictive Disorders" in Chapter 6.)

Minutes 18–23

Past Medical History

"Do you have any chronic medical problems? Have these illnesses affected you emotionally? Have you ever undergone surgery? Have you ever experienced a seizure or hit your head so hard that you lost consciousness? Do you take any medications for medical illness? Do you take any supplements, vitamins, or over-the-counter or herbal medicines regularly?"

Allergies. *"Are you allergic to any medications? Can you describe your allergy?"*

Family history. *"Have any of your relatives ever had mental or behavioral health problems, such as attention-deficit/hyperactivity disorder, anxiety, depression, bipolar disorder, psychosis, problems from drinking or drugs, suicide attempts, nervous breakdowns, or psychiatric hospitalizations?"*

Developmental history. *"Do you know if your mother had any difficulties during her pregnancy or delivery? What were you like as a young child? Did you ever receive developmental, speech, or special education services?"* (See Chapter 12, "Developmental Milestones," for early developmental milestones.) Look at the child's current height and weight on a growth curve.

Social history. *"Did you have any behavior or learning problems during your early childhood? When you started school, did* you have trouble relating socially to your classmates or difficulty keeping up academically? How far have you made it in school? Who lived in your home during your early childhood? Who lives there now? Was a religious faith part of your upbringing? Currently? Have you ever held a job outside of the home? Have you ever been suspended? Expelled? Arrested? Jailed? What do you like to do? How do you spend your time online? What do you like about yourself? What do your friends like about you? Do you have any friends you can confide in? Are you sexually active? Are you really uncomfortable with your assigned gender?"

Minutes 24–28

Mental Status Examination

By this point of the interview, you should have already observed or obtained most of the pertinent mental status examination data. See Chapter 9, "The Mental Status Examination: A Psychiatric Glossary," for a more detailed version of the mental status examination, which includes the following components:

- Appearance
- Behavior
- Speech
- Emotion
- Thought process
- Thought content
- Cognition and intellectual resources
- Insight and judgment: *"What problems do you have? Are you sick in any way? What are your future plans?"*

Mini-Mental State Examination

The Mini-Mental State Examination (MMSE) is a commonly used basic cognition ability assessment in adult and geriatric psychiatric care that has standardized questions and yields a numerical score. We find that the MMSE is less pertinent to administer to young persons than to older adults. When it is used, the MMSE is more challenging to interpret for the younger developmental ages. However, if a major mental illness (e.g., schizophrenia) or encephalopathy is suspected, a MMSE may add diagnostic value. When the MMSE is used, the lead-in could be along the lines of *"Have you had any prob-*

lems with your concentration or your memory? Can you help me understand the extent to which you might be having those types of difficulties?" The MMSE then includes the following items: name, date and time, place, immediate recall, attention (counting backward from 100 by 7s, spelling *world* backward), delayed recall, general information (president, governor, five large cities), abstractions, proverbs, naming, repetition, three-stage command, reading, copying, and writing (Folstein et al. 1975).

Minutes 29–30

Ask any follow-up questions. Thank the patient for her time and, if appropriate, begin discussing diagnosis and treatment.

Consider asking the following: *"Have the questions I asked addressed your major concerns? Is there anything important I missed or anything that I really should know about to better understand what you are going through?"*

SECTION II

Using DSM-5 With Children and Adolescents

Chapter 6

DSM-5 Pediatric Diagnostic Interview

In Chapter 5, "The 30-Minute Pediatric Diagnostic Interview," we outlined a diagnostic interview that included a screening question for each of the DSM-5 (American Psychiatric Association 2013) categories of mental disorders commonly experienced by children and adolescents. If you are speaking with a young person who answers affirmatively to one of those questions, we show how the screening questions are the avenues of the psychiatric diagnostic interview. A good interviewer skillfully travels these avenues with a young person and, when possible, reaches a specific and accurate diagnosis along the way.

This chapter follows the order of DSM-5 disorder categories, beginning with neurodevelopmental disorders. For each category of DSM-5 diagnoses presented, whether bipolar disorders or elimination disorders, the section begins with one or more screening questions from the model interview presented in Chapter 5. After the screening questions, follow-up questions are provided. If the follow-up questions include a measure of impairment or a measure of time, these measures are a required part of the subsequent diagnostic criteria. By asking follow-up questions before the additional symptom questions in the diagnostic criteria, we make the interview more efficient and precise while reserving the full diagnosis of a mental disorder for a person impaired by his experiences.

The screening and follow-up questions are followed by the diagnostic criteria. When the diagnostic criteria are to be elicited by the interviewer, we offer italicized prompts for the relevant symptom. We structured these questions so that an affirmative answer meets the criteria for that symptom. When the diagnostic criteria are observed rather than elicited, as in the case of disorganized speech, psychomotor retardation, or autonomic hyperactivity, they are listed as instructions to the interviewer, set in roman type. The minimum number of symptoms necessary to reach a particular diagnosis is underlined. We do not list all the possible questions that can be used to elicit a relevant symptom, but the included questions are specifically designed to follow DSM-5. To make the diagnostic process as clear as possible, we have included negative criteria for a DSM-5 diagnosis under the heading "Exclusion(s)." For example, DSM-5 observes that a young person's recurrent, aggressive outbursts do not meet criteria for intermittent explosive disorder if they occur only during an adjustment disorder. These exclusion criteria usually do not require you to ask a specific question but instead depend on the history you elicit. The most common subtypes, specifiers, and severity measures are listed under the heading "Modifiers," but the complete array of modifiers is found only in DSM-5.

In the interest of brevity, this guide includes diagnostic questions for the most common DSM-5 disorders. The idea is to focus on learning the diagnostic criteria for the paradigmatic disorders in each section before exploring the related diagnoses—that is, to know the main streets of DSM-5 before learning its side streets.

In this book, the side streets are labeled as *alternatives*, a term that is not used in DSM-5. These alternatives include only related diagnoses from the same DSM-5 chapter. For example, schizophreniform disorder is listed as an alternative to schizophrenia because both are grouped together in DSM-5. In contrast, bipolar I disorder and other diagnoses listed in the differential diagnosis for schizophrenia are not in the alternatives section for schizophrenia because the disorders are found in different sections of DSM-5. For each diagnosis listed as alternatives, the essential diagnostic criteria are included, and the interviewer is referred to the corresponding pages in DSM-5 to read the diagnostic criteria and associated material in detail.

We eliminated repetitive DSM-5 criteria, especially for the various mental disorders associated with another medical condition or substance-induced mental disorders, in which, broadly, the symptoms of a disorder are present as a direct effect of another medical condition or the use of a substance.

As this overview suggests, this book is not a substitute for DSM-5 but serves as a practical diagnostic tool with specific phrasing you can use, an operationalized version of DSM-5—the equivalent of the sketched version of a city street that a GPS device displays rather than the detailed portrait of each side street. If you desire those details, after each diagnosis we list a series of numbers and a letter that direct you to additional information. For example, after autism spectrum disorder, you will see this notation: [F84.0, 50–59].

The first entry is the ICD-10 (World Health Organization 1992) code, and the second entry is the page numbers of the main DSM-5 text for the disorder. These codes and references are provided to assist practitioners with coding and with quickly finding additional information.

Unfortunately, at times, the notations are more cryptic, as in this notation: [F90.x, 59–65].

As before, the first entry is the ICD-10 code corresponding to attention-deficit/hyperactivity disorder, and the second entry is the page numbers of the main DSM-5 text for the disorder. However, the use of an "x" indicates that you need additional information to find the specific ICD-10 code. In this case, that additional information is whether a young person's deficits are predominantly inattentive, predominantly hyperactive/impulsive, or a combined presentation, which can be found in the specifiers section following the main diagnostic criteria. We organized the diagnoses this way to reduce the repetitive listing of diagnoses and to keep your focus on efficient, accurate diagnoses. ICD-10 codes are complex. (The ICD is, after all, a diagnostic list that includes codes for being struck by an orca, an exceedingly uncommon event.) Listing every code would double the length of this book, which would reduce its clinical utility. Listing every code would also shift the focus of the book to accurate coding, whereas our goal is to help you make an accurate diagnosis.

As this strategy suggests, we tried to balance brevity and detail. For each diagnosis, the notation always provides the general form of the ICD-10 codes, along with the page numbers of DSM-5 so that you can quickly find the additional information you need. This book lacks the rich detail of DSM-5 but will deliver you to your diagnostic destination in a timely fashion.

Neurodevelopmental Disorders

DSM-5 pp. 31–86

This section contains questions phrased for interviewing an older child with an ability to self-reflect. For younger children, rephrase these questions to interview the child's caregiver instead.

Screening questions: *Did you have any learning problems, or did you get into trouble a lot for your behavior when you were younger? When you started school, did you have trouble getting along with your classmates or difficulty keeping up academically?*

   If yes, ask: *Do you have trouble concentrating or struggle with being impulsive or overactive? Do you have difficulty communicating with other people? Are there specific things that you do frequently and find hard to control? Do you struggle to learn, more than your classmates do?*

- If deficits in intellectual functioning or specific academic skills predominate, proceed to intellectual disability (intellectual developmental disorder) criteria.
- If deficits in social interactions or impairing motor behaviors predominate, proceed to autism spectrum disorder criteria.
- If inattention, hyperactivity, or impulsivity predominate, proceed to attention-deficit/hyperactivity disorder criteria.

1. Intellectual Disability (Intellectual Developmental Disorder) [F7x, 33–41]

   a. Inclusion: Requires intellectual deficits, beginning during early development, that impair adaptive function as manifested by <u>both</u> of the following symptoms.

      i. Deficits in intellectual functions, such as reasoning, problem solving, planning, abstract thinking, judgment, academic learning, and experiential learning. Must be confirmed by both clinical assessment and individualized, standardized intelligence testing.

      ii. Impaired adaptive functioning, normalized for age and culture, which restricts participation and performance in one or more aspects of daily life activities. The limitations result in the need for ongoing support at school, at work, or for independent life.

   b. Modifiers

      i. Severity (DSM-5, pp. 34–36, Table 1)
         - Mild (F70, 34)
         - Moderate (F71, 35)
         - Severe (F72, 36)
         - Profound (F73, 36)

c. Alternatives

    i. If a person younger than 5 years fails to meet expected developmental milestones in several areas of intellectual functioning and is unable to undergo systematic assessment of intellectual functioning, consider global developmental delay [F88, 41], a diagnosis that requires reassessment after a period of time.

    ii. If a person older than 5 years has intellectual disability that cannot be well characterized because of associated sensory or physical impairments, consider unspecified intellectual disability (intellectual developmental disorder) [F79, 41], a diagnosis that requires eventual reassessment and should be reserved for exceptional circumstances.

    iii. If a person has persistent difficulties in the acquisition of language (spoken, written, sign, or other modalities) that begin in the early developmental period and result in substantial functional limitations, consider the diagnosis of language disorder [F80.2, 42–44]. Language disorders occur as a primary impairment or coexist with other disorders. This diagnosis should not be used if the language difficulties are better explained by hearing or sensory impairment, intellectual disability, or global developmental delay or are caused by another medical or neurological condition.

    iv. If a person has persistent difficulties in speech sound production that interfere with speech intelligibility or prevent verbal communication of messages, consider speech sound disorder [F80.0, 44–45]. The symptoms must be present in the early developmental period and result in limitations in effective communication, social participation, academic achievement, and occupational performance, individually or in any combination. Speech sound disorder occurs as a primary impairment or coexists with other disorders or congenital or acquired conditions. This diagnosis should not be used if the speech sound difficulties are due to congenital or acquired medical or neurological conditions.

    v. If a person has marked and frequent disturbances in the fluency and time patterning of speech that are inappropriate for the person's age and language skills, consider childhood-onset fluency disorder (stuttering) [F80.81, 45–47]. Symptoms must begin in the early developmental period. The disturbance must cause anxiety about speaking or the ability to communicate effectively. This disorder co-occurs with other disorders. The diagnosis should not be used if the disorder is attributable to a speech-motor or sensory deficit, is due to another medical or neurological condition, or is better explained by another mental disorder.

vi. If a person has persistent difficulties in the social use of verbal and nonverbal communication that functionally limit effective communication, social participation, social relationships, academic achievement, or occupational performance, consider social (pragmatic) communication disorder [F80.89, 47–49]. Symptoms begin during the early developmental period. This disorder co-occurs with other disorders. The diagnosis should not be used if the symptoms are better explained by intellectual disability, global developmental delay, or another mental disorder or are attributable to another medical or neurological condition.

vii. If a person has symptoms of a communication disorder that cause clinically significant distress or impairment but do not meet the full criteria for a communication disorder or another neurodevelopmental disorder, consider unspecified communication disorder [F80.9, 49].

viii. If a person has persistent difficulties in learning and using academic skills that begin during school-age years and eventually result in significant interference with academic or occupational performance, consider specific learning disorder [F81.x, 66–74]. To meet criteria, the current skills must be well below the average range for the person's age, gender, cultural group, and level of education. The symptoms must not be better accounted for by another intellectual, medical, mental, neurological, or sensory disorder.

2. Autism Spectrum Disorder [F84.0, 50–59]

This section contains questions phrased for interviewing an older child with an ability to self-reflect. For younger children or those with limited cognitive functioning, rephrase these questions to interview the child's caregiver instead.

a. Inclusion: Requires persistent deficits in social communication and social interaction, across multiple contexts, that are present in early childhood but that may not be manifest until social demands exceed limited capacities and that cause clinically significant impairment in functioning. The disorder is marked by <u>all</u> of the following persistent deficits in social communication and interaction.

   i. Deficits in social-emotional reciprocity: *How do you introduce yourself to other people? Do you find it hard to greet another person? Do you find it hard to share your interests, thoughts, and feelings with other people? Do you dislike hearing about what other people are interested in or how they feel?*

   ii. Deficits in nonverbal communicative behaviors used for social interaction; these are usually observed by a practitioner and range from poorly integrated verbal and nonverbal communication, to abnormalities in eye contact and body language or deficits in understanding and use of nonverbal communication, to total lack of facial expression or gestures.

   iii. Deficits in developing and maintaining relationships: *Are you disinterested in other people? Are you unable to engage in imaginative play with other people? Do you find it difficult to make new friends? When a situation changes, do you find it hard to adjust what you do in response?*

b. Inclusion: In addition, the diagnosis requires at least <u>two</u> of the following signs of restricted, repetitive patterns of behavior, interests, or activities.

   i. Stereotyped or repetitive speech, motor movements, or use of objects, such as simple motor stereotypies, echolalia, repetitive use of objects, or idiosyncratic phrases.

   ii. Insistence on sameness and excessive adherence to routines or avoidance of change: *Do you have any special routines or patterns of behavior? What happens when you cannot follow these routines or engage in these behaviors? Do you struggle to change?*

      iii.   Restricted interests of abnormal intensity or focus: *Do you intensely focus on, or find yourself very interested in, just a few things?*

      iv.   Hyper- or hyporeactivity to sensory input: *Do you have intense responses to something that is painful? Something hot? Something cold? Are there particular sounds, textures, or smells to which you respond strongly? Do you find yourself fascinated with lights or spinning objects?*

c. Modifiers

    i.   Specifiers

- With (or without) accompanying intellectual impairment
- With (or without) accompanying language impairment
- Associated with a known medical or genetic condition or environmental factor
- Associated with another neurodevelopmental, mental, or behavioral disorder
- With catatonia

    ii.   Severity is coded separately for the social communication impairments and for the restricted, repetitive patterns of behavior.

- Level 1: Requiring support
- Level 2: Requiring substantial support
- Level 3: Requiring very substantial support

d. Alternatives

    i.   If a person shows motor performance substantially below expected levels, which significantly interferes with activities of daily living or academic achievement, consider developmental coordination disorder [F82, 74–77]. Examples include clumsiness, as well as slow and inaccurate performance of motor skills. The disturbance cannot be due to another medical or neurological condition or be better explained by another mental disorder.

    ii.   If a person has repetitive, seemingly driven, yet apparently purposeless motor behavior, such as hand shaking or waving, body rocking, head banging, or self-biting, consider stereotypic movement disorder [F98.4, 77–80]. The motor disturbance causes clinically significant distress or impairment. The motor behavior is not due to the direct physiological effects of a substance or a general medical condition and is not better explained by the symptoms of another mental disorder.

iii. A tic is a sudden, rapid, recurrent, nonrhythmic motor movement or vocalization. If a person experiences both motor and vocal tics beginning before age 18 years, consider Tourette's disorder [F95.2, 81–85]. The tics may wax and wane in frequency but must persist for at least 1 year after onset. The tics cannot be due to the direct physiological effects of another medical condition or a substance.

iv. If a person experiences either motor or vocal tics, but not both, during his illness, and has never met criteria for Tourette's disorder, consider persistent (chronic) motor or vocal tic disorder [F95.1, 81–85]. The onset is before age 18 years, and the tics may wax and wane in frequency but must have persisted for more than 1 year since their onset.

v. If a person experiences motor and/or vocal tics for less than 1 year, beginning before age 18 years, and the tics are not due to the direct physiological consequences of a substance or another medical condition, and he has never met criteria for Tourette's disorder or persistent (chronic) motor or vocal tic disorder, consider provisional tic disorder [F95.0, 81–85].

vi. If a person experiences tics that do not meet criteria for a specific tic disorder because the movements or vocalizations are atypical in relation to age at onset or clinical presentation, consider other specified tic disorder [F95.8, 85] or unspecified tic disorder [F95.9, 85].

3. Attention-Deficit/Hyperactivity Disorder [F90.x, 59–65]

a. Inclusion: Requires a pattern of behavior, with onset before age 12 years, that is present in multiple settings and gives rise to social, educational, or work performance difficulties. The symptoms must be persistently present for at least 6 months to a degree inconsistent with developmental level. The disorder is manifested by at least six of the following symptoms of inattention.

i. Overlooks details: *Over at least the last 6 months, have other people told you that you often overlook or miss details or that you made careless mistakes in your work?*

ii. Task inattention: *Do you often have difficulty staying focused on a task or an activity, such as reading a lengthy text or listening to a lecture or conversation?*

iii. Appears not to listen: *Do other people tell you that when they speak to you, your mind often seems to be elsewhere or that it seems like you are not listening?*

iv. Fails to finish tasks: *Do you often struggle to finish schoolwork, chores, or work assignments because you lose focus or are easily sidetracked?*

v. Difficulty organizing tasks: *Do you often find it difficult to organize tasks or activities? Do you struggle with time management or fail to meet deadlines?*

vi. Avoids tasks requiring sustained mental activity: *Do you often avoid tasks that require sustained focus?*

vii. Often loses things necessary for tasks: *Do you often lose things that are essential for tasks or activities, such as school materials, books, tools, wallets, keys, paperwork, eyeglasses, or your phone?*

viii. Easily distracted: *Do you find that you are often easily distracted by things or thoughts unrelated to the activity or task you are supposed to be doing?*

ix. Often forgetful: *Do you find, or do other people find, that you are often forgetful in your daily activities?*

b. Inclusion: Alternatively, requires the presence of at least <u>six</u> of the following manifestations of hyperactivity and impulsivity over the same course.

i. Fidgets: *Over the last 6 months, have you often found yourself fidgeting with your hands or feet? Do you find it hard to sit without squirming?*

ii. Leaves seat: *When you are in a situation where you are expected to sit, do you often leave your seat?*

iii. Runs or climbs: *Do you often find yourself running around or climbing in a situation where doing so is inappropriate?*

iv. Unable to maintain quiet: *Do you often find yourself unable to work or play quietly?*

v. Hyperactivity: *Do you often feel as if you are, or do other people describe you as always being, "on the go" or as acting as if you were "driven by a motor?" Is it hard to sit still for an extended time?*

vi. Talks excessively: *Do you often talk excessively?*

vii. Blurts answers: *Do you often struggle to wait your turn in a conversation? Do you often complete other people's sentences or blurt out an answer before a question has been completed?*

    viii. Struggles to take turns: *Do you often have difficulty waiting your turn or waiting in line?*

    ix. Interrupts or intrudes: *Do you often butt into other people's activities, conversations, or games? Do you often start using other people's things without permission?*

c. Exclusion: If the criteria are not met in two or more settings or there is no evidence that the symptoms interfere with functioning, the symptoms occur only in the context of a psychotic disorder, or the symptoms are better explained by another mental disorder, do not use this diagnosis.

d. Modifiers

    i. Specifiers

- Combined presentation [F90.2, 60]: If both inattention and hyperactivity-impulsivity criteria are met for the past 6 months.
- Predominantly inattentive presentation [F90.0, 60]: If inattention criteria are met but hyperactivity-impulsivity criteria have not been met for the past 6 months.
- Predominantly hyperactive/impulsive presentation [F90.1, 60]: If hyperactivity-impulsivity criteria are met and inattention criteria have not been met for the past 6 months.
- In partial remission if full criteria no longer met but still symptomatic.

    ii. Severity

- Mild: Few, if any, symptoms in excess of those required to make the diagnosis are present, and symptoms result in no more than minor impairments in social or occupational functioning.
- Moderate: Symptoms or functional impairment between "mild" and "severe" is present.
- Severe: Many symptoms in excess of those required to make the diagnosis, or several symptoms that are particularly severe, are present, or the symptoms result in marked impairment in social or occupational functioning.

e. Alternatives: If a young person is experiencing sub-threshold symptoms or you have not yet had sufficient opportunity to verify all criteria, consider other speci-fied attention-deficit/hyperactivity disorder [F90.8, 65–66] or unspecified attention-deficit/hyperactivity disor-der [F90.9, 66]. The symptoms must be associated with impairment and do not occur exclusively during the course of schizophrenia or another psychotic disorder and are not better explained by another mental disorder.

Schizophrenia Spectrum and Other Psychotic Disorders

DSM-5 pp. 87–122

Screening questions: *Have you seen visions or other things that other people did not see? Have you heard noises, sounds, or voices that other people did not hear? Do you ever feel as if people are fol-lowing you or trying to hurt you in some way? Have you ever felt that you had special powers or found special messages from the ra-dio or TV seemingly meant just for you?*

    If yes, ask: *Do these experiences change what you do or tell you to do things? Did these experiences ever cause you significant trouble with your friends or family, at school, or in another setting?*

• If yes, proceed to schizophrenia criteria.

1. Schizophrenia [F20.9, 99–105]

   a. Inclusion: Requires at least 6 months of continuous signs of disturbance, which may include prodromal or residual symptoms. During at least 1 month of that period, at least <u>two</u> of the following symptoms are present, and at least <u>one</u> of the symptoms must be de-lusions, hallucinations, or disorganized speech.

       i. Delusions: *Is anyone working to harm or hurt you? When you read a book, watch television, or work at a com-puter, do you ever find that there are messages intended just for you? Do you have special powers or abilities?*

       ii. Hallucinations: *When you are awake, do you ever hear a voice different from your own thoughts that other peo-ple cannot hear? When you are awake, do you ever see things that other people cannot see?*

     iii. Disorganized speech such as frequent derailment or incoherence

     iv. Grossly disorganized or catatonic behavior

     v. Negative symptoms such as diminished emotional expression or avolition

b. Exclusions

     i. If the disturbance is attributable to the physiological effects of a substance (e.g., a drug of abuse, a medication) or another medical condition, do not use this diagnosis.

     ii. If a young person has been diagnosed with an autism spectrum disorder, schizophrenia may be diagnosed only if prominent delusions or hallucinations are also present for at least 1 month.

c. Modifiers

     i. Specifiers

- First episode, currently in acute episode
- First episode, currently in partial remission
- First episode, currently in full remission
- Multiple episodes, currently in acute episode
- Multiple episodes, currently in partial remission
- Multiple episodes, currently in full remission
- Continuous
- Unspecified

     ii. Additional specifiers

- With catatonia [F06.1, 119–120]: Use when at least <u>three</u> of the following are present: catalepsy, waxy flexibility, stupor, agitation, mutism, negativism, posturing, mannerisms, stereotypies, grimacing, echolalia, echopraxia.

     iii. Severity

- Severity is rated by a quantitative assessment of the primary symptoms of psychosis, each of which may be rated for its current severity on a five-point scale (see Clinician-Rated Dimensions of Psychosis Symptom Severity in DSM-5, pp. 743–744).

d. Alternatives

     i. If a person experiences only delusions, whether bizarre or nonbizarre; has never met full criteria for schizophrenia; and has functioning that is not markedly impaired beyond the ramifications of his delusion, consider delusional disorder [F22, 90–93]. The criteria include multiple specifiers. The diagnosis should not be used if the delusions are due to the physiological effects of a substance or another medical condition. The diagnosis also should not be used if the delusions are better explained by another mental disorder.

ii. If a person has experienced at least 1 day but less than 1 month of schizophrenia symptoms, consider brief psychotic disorder [F23, 94–96]. The person usually has an acute onset, fewer negative symptoms, and less functional impairment and always experiences an eventual return to the previous level of functioning.

iii. If a person has experienced at least 1 month but less than 6 months of schizophrenia symptoms, consider schizophreniform disorder [F20.81, 96–99]. The criteria include specifiers for catatonia, as well as with and without good prognostic features.

iv. If a person who meets criteria for schizophrenia also experiences major mood disturbances—either major depressive episodes or manic episodes—for at least half the time he has met criteria for schizophrenia, consider schizoaffective disorder [F25.x, 105–110]. Over a person's lifetime, he also must have experienced at least 2 weeks of delusions or hallucinations in the absence of a major mood episode.

v. If a substance or medication directly causes a psychotic episode, consider substance/medication-induced psychotic disorder [F1x.x, 110–115].

vi. If another medical condition directly causes the psychotic episode, consider psychotic disorder due to another medical condition [F06.x, 115–118].

vii. If a person experiences psychotic symptoms that cause clinically significant distress or functional impairment without meeting full criteria for another psychotic disorder, consider unspecified schizophrenia spectrum and other psychotic disorder [F29, 122]. To communicate the specific reason a person's symptoms do not meet the criteria, consider other specified schizophrenia spectrum and other psychotic disorder [F28, 122]. Examples include persistent auditory hallucinations in the absence of any other psychotic symptom and delusional symptoms in the partner of an individual with delusional disorder.

Bipolar and Related Disorders

DSM-5 pp. 123–154

Screening question: *Has there been a time when for many days straight your mood was super happy, you were more self-confident, and you had much more energy than usual?*

If yes, ask: *During those times, did you feel this way all day or most of the day? Did something happen that started those feelings? Did those times ever last at least a week or result in your being hospitalized? Did these periods ever cause you significant trouble with your friends or family, at school, or in another setting?*

- If symptoms lasted a week or caused hospitalization, proceed to bipolar I disorder criteria.
- If not, proceed to bipolar II disorder criteria.

1. Bipolar I Disorder [F31.x, 123–132]

For a diagnosis of bipolar I disorder, it is necessary to meet criteria for at least one manic episode. The manic episode may have been preceded by and may be followed by hypomanic episodes or major depressive episodes.

a. Inclusion: A manic episode—defined as a distinct period of abnormally and persistently elevated or irritable mood and increased goal-directed activity or energy, lasting at least 1 week and present most of the day—requires at least **three** of the following symptoms.

i. Inflated self-esteem or grandiosity: *During that period, did you feel especially confident, as though you could accomplish something extraordinary that you could not have done otherwise?*

ii. Decreased need for sleep: *During that period, did you notice any change in how much sleep you needed to feel rested? Did you feel rested after less than 3 hours of sleep?*

iii. More talkative than usual: *During that period, did anyone tell you that you talked more than usual or that it was hard to interrupt you?*

    iv. Flight of ideas: *During that period, were your thoughts racing? Did you have so many ideas that you could not keep up with them?*

    v. Distractibility: *During that period, were you having more trouble than usual focusing? Did you find yourself easily distracted?*

    vi. Increased goal-directed activity: *During that period, how did you spend your time? Did you find yourself much more active than usual?*

    vii. Excessive involvement in activities that have a high potential for painful consequences: *During that period, did you engage in activities that were unusual for you? Did you spend money, use substances, or engage in sexual activities in a way that is unusual for you? Did any of these activities cause trouble for anyone?*

b. Exclusions

    i. The occurrence of manic or major depressive episode(s) is not better explained by schizoaffective disorder, schizophrenia, schizophreniform disorder, delusional disorder, or other specified or unspecified schizophrenia spectrum and other psychotic disorder.

    ii. The episode is not due to the physiological effects of a substance or another medical condition. However, a manic episode that both emerges during antidepressant treatment *and* persists beyond the physiological effect of the treatment meets criteria for bipolar I disorder.

c. Modifiers

    i. Current (or most recent) episode

- Manic [F31.x, 126–127]
- Hypomanic
- Depressed [F31.x, 126–127]
- Unspecified (use when the symptoms, but not the duration, of an episode meet criteria)

    ii. Specifiers

- With anxious distress
- With mixed features: Use if at least <u>three</u> of the symptoms of a major depressive episode are present simultaneously.
- With rapid cycling

- With melancholic features
- With atypical features
- With mood-congruent psychotic features
- With mood-incongruent psychotic features
- With catatonia
- With peripartum onset
- With seasonal pattern

   iii. Course and severity

- Current or most recent episode manic, hypomanic, depressed, unspecified
  - Mild, moderate, severe
  - With psychotic features
  - In partial remission, in full remission
  - Unspecified

  d. Alternatives

   i. If a substance directly causes the episode, including a substance prescribed to treat depression, consider substance/medication-induced bipolar and related disorder [F1x.xx, 142–145].

   ii. If another medical condition causes the episode, consider bipolar and related disorder due to another medical condition [F06.3x, 145–147].

2. Bipolar II Disorder [F31.81, 132–139]

For a diagnosis of bipolar II disorder, it is necessary to meet criteria for at least one hypomanic episode. The hypomanic episode may have been preceded by and may be followed by major depressive episodes.

  a. Inclusion: A hypomanic episode—defined as a distinct period of abnormally and persistently elevated or irritable mood and increased goal-directed activity or energy, lasting at least 4 days and present most of the day—requires the presence of at least three of the following symptoms.

   i. Inflated self-esteem or grandiosity: *During that period, did you feel especially confident, as though you could accomplish something extraordinary that you could not have done otherwise?*

   ii. Decreased need for sleep: *During that period, did you notice any change in how much sleep you needed to feel rested? Did you feel rested after less than 3 hours of sleep?*

    iii. More talkative than usual: *During that period, did anyone tell you that you talked more than usual or that it was hard to interrupt you?*

    iv. Flight of ideas: *During that period, were your thoughts racing? Did you have so many ideas that you could not keep up with them?*

    v. Distractibility: *During that period, were you having more trouble than usual focusing? Did you find yourself easily distracted?*

    vi. Increased goal-directed activity: *During that period, how did you spend your time? Did you find yourself much more active than usual?*

    vii. Excessive involvement in activities that have a high potential for painful consequences: *During that period, did you engage in activities that were unusual for you? Did you spend money, use substances, or engage in sexual activities in a way that is unusual for you? Did any of these activities cause trouble for anyone?*

b. Exclusions

    i. If there has ever been a manic episode or if the episode is attributable to the physiological effects of a substance/medication, do not use this diagnosis.

    ii. If the hypomanic episode is better explained by schizoaffective disorder, schizophrenia, schizophreniform disorder, delusional disorder, or other specified or unspecified schizophrenia spectrum and other psychotic disorders, do not use this diagnosis.

    iii. If the hypomanic episode is severe enough to cause marked impairment in social or occupational functioning or to necessitate hospitalization, do not use this diagnosis.

c. Modifiers

    i. Specify current or most recent episode

- Hypomanic
- Depressed

    ii. Specifiers

- With anxious distress
- With mixed features: Use if at least <u>three</u> of the symptoms of a major depressive episode are present simultaneously.
- With rapid cycling
- With mood-congruent psychotic features

- With mood-incongruent psychotic features
- With catatonia
- With peripartum onset
- With seasonal pattern

iii. Course

- In partial remission
- In full remission

iv. Severity

- Mild
- Moderate
- Severe

d. Alternatives

i. If a person reports 1 or more years of multiple hypomanic and depressive symptoms that never rose to the level of a hypomanic or major depressive episode, consider cyclothymic disorder [F34.0, 139–141]. During the same 1-year period, the hypomanic and depressive periods have been present for at least half the time, and the individual has not been without the symptoms for more than 2 months at a time. If the symptoms are due to the physiological effects of a substance or another medical condition, do not use this diagnosis.

ii. If a person experiences symptoms characteristic of bipolar disorder that cause clinically significant distress or functional impairment without meeting full criteria for a bipolar disorder, consider unspecified bipolar and related disorder [F31.9, 149–154]. To communicate the specific reason a person's symptoms do not meet the criteria, as in short-duration hypomania, short-duration cyclothymia, and hypomania without prior major depressive episode, consider other specified bipolar and related disorder [F31.89, 148].

Depressive Disorders

DSM-5 pp. 155–188

Screening question: *Have you been feeling sad, blue, down, depressed, or irritable? If so, does feeling this way make it hard to do things, to concentrate, or to sleep? Are you angry most of the time?*

If yes, ask: *Did those times ever last at least 2 weeks? Did these periods ever cause you significant trouble with your friends or family, at school, or in another setting?*

- If yes, proceed to major depressive disorder criteria.
- If a child age 6 years or older says no, ask the irritability screening question, which appears after the specifiers for major depressive disorder later in this section.

1. Major Depressive Disorder [F3x.xx, 160–168]

   a. Inclusion: Requires the presence of at least <u>five</u> of the following symptoms, which must include either depressed mood or loss of interest or pleasure (anhedonia), during the same 2-week episode.

      i. Depressed mood most of the day (already assessed)
      ii. Markedly diminished interest or pleasure in activities (already assessed)
      iii. Significant weight loss or gain: *During that period, did you notice any change in your appetite? Did you notice any change in your weight?*
      iv. Insomnia or hypersomnia: *During that period, how much and how well were you sleeping?*
      v. Psychomotor agitation or retardation: *During that period, did anyone tell you that you seemed to move faster or slower than usual?*
      vi. Fatigue or loss of energy: *During that period, what was your energy level like? Did anyone tell you that you seemed worn down or less energetic than usual?*
      vii. Feelings of worthlessness or excessive guilt: *During that period, did you feel tremendous regret or guilt about current or past events or relationships?*
      viii. Diminished concentration: *During that period, were you able to make decisions or concentrate like you usually do?*
      ix. Recurrent thoughts of death or suicide: *During that period, did you think about death more than you usually do? Have you thought about hurting yourself or taking your own life?*

   b. Exclusions

      i. If there has ever been a manic episode or a hypomanic episode, or the major depressive episode is attributable to the physiological effects of a substance or to another medical condition, do not use this diagnosis.

   ii. If the major depressive episode is better explained by schizoaffective disorder, schizophrenia, schizophreniform disorder, delusional disorder, or other specified and unspecified schizophrenia spectrum and other psychotic disorders, do not use this diagnosis.

c. Modifiers

   i. Specifiers

   - With anxious distress
   - With mixed features: Use if at least <u>three</u> of the symptoms of a major depressive episode are present simultaneously.
   - With melancholic features
   - With atypical features
   - With mood-congruent psychotic features
   - With mood-incongruent psychotic features
   - With catatonia
   - With peripartum onset
   - With seasonal pattern

   ii. Course and severity

   - Single episode
   - Recurrent episode
   - Mild [F3x.0, 162]
   - Moderate [F3x.1, 162]
   - Severe [F3x.2, 162]
   - With psychotic features [F3x.3, 162]
   - In partial remission [F3x.4, 162]
   - In full remission [F3x.xx, 162]
   - Unspecified [F3x.9, 162]

d. Alternatives

   i. If a person reports experiencing depression or anhedonia for at least 1 year resulting in clinically significant distress or impairment, along with at least <u>two</u> of the symptoms of a major depressive episode, consider persistent depressive disorder (dysthymia) [F34.1, 168–171]. If a person experiences 2 continuous months without depressive symptoms, do not use this diagnosis. If the person has ever had symptoms that met the criteria for a bipolar disorder or a cyclothymic disorder, do not use this diagnosis. If the disturbance is better explained by a psychotic disorder or is due to the physiological effects of a substance or another medical condition, do not use this diagnosis.

ii. If a young woman describes pronounced mood changes that begin in the week before her menses, decrease in the week after menses, and abate in the week postmenses, consider premenstrual dysphoric disorder [N94.3, 171–175]. The diagnostic criteria include at least <u>one</u> of the following: marked affective lability, marked irritability or interpersonal conflicts, marked depressed mood, or marked anxiety. At least <u>one</u> of the following symptoms must additionally be present (to reach a total of <u>five</u> symptoms when combined with the symptoms above): decreased interest in usual activities; subjective difficulty in concentration; lethargy, easy fatigability, or marked lack of energy; change in appetite; hypersomnia or insomnia; sense of being overwhelmed; or physical symptoms such as breast tenderness or swelling, joint or muscle pain, bloating, and weight gain.

iii. If a substance directly causes the episode, including a substance prescribed to treat depression, consider a substance/medication-induced depressive disorder [F1x.x4, 175–180].

iv. If another medical condition causes the episode, consider a depressive disorder due to another medical condition [F06.3x, 180–183].

v. If a person experiences a depressive episode that causes clinically significant distress or functional impairment without meeting full criteria for a depressive disorder, consider unspecified depressive disorder [F32.9, 184]. To communicate the specific reason a young person's symptoms do not meet the criteria, consider other specified depressive disorder [F32.8, 183–184]. Examples includes recurrent brief depression and depressive episode with insufficient symptoms.

Irritability screening question for children older than 6 years: *Do you lose your temper, get mad, and yell or hit things?*

If yes, ask: *Do you lose your temper and feel really mad every day or every other day? Does your angry mood or yelling cause trouble at home or school?*

- If yes, proceed to disruptive mood dysregulation disorder criteria.
- If no, seek collateral information from caregivers or proceed to another diagnostic category.

2. Disruptive Mood Dysregulation Disorder [F34.8, 156–160]

   a. Inclusion: Requires severe recurrent temper outbursts in response to common stressors, averaging at least three per week, for at least 1 year. The outbursts must occur in at least two distinct settings such as school or home, be severe in at least one setting, begin before age 10 years but not before age 6 years, and be characterized by the following <u>three</u> symptoms.

      i. Temper or behavioral outbursts: *When you get upset or lose your temper, what happens? Do you yell? Do you slap, punch, bite, or hit another person? Do you break or destroy things?*

      ii. Disproportionate reaction: *When you get upset or lose your temper, do you know what sets you off? What kinds of things bother you so much that you feel like yelling or hitting?*

      iii. Persistently irritable of angry mood between temper outbursts: *When you are not yelling or upset, how do you feel inside? Do you usually feel grouchy, angry, irritable, or sad?*

   b. Exclusions

      i. These responses must be inconsistent with a child's developmental level.

      ii. If the behaviors occur exclusively during an episode of major depressive disorder and are better explained by another mental disorder (e.g., autism spectrum disorder, posttraumatic stress disorder, separation anxiety disorder, persistent depressive disorder [dysthymia]), do not use this diagnosis.

      iii. If the symptoms are attributable to the physiological effects of a substance or to another medical or neurological condition, do not use this diagnosis.

      iv. If a child is currently diagnosed with oppositional defiant disorder, intermittent explosive disorder, or bipolar disorder, do not use this diagnosis.

c. Alternatives: If, during the last year, there was a period lasting at least 1 day during which the child had abnormally elevated mood and <u>three</u> criteria of a manic episode, consider the possibility of a bipolar disorder (see DSM-5, pp. 123–154).

Anxiety Disorders

<u>DSM-5 pp. 189–233</u>

Screening question: *Would you say that you worry a lot or more than other kids your age? Do people say that you worry too much or are too shy? Do you feel afraid when you're alone or away from your family? Do you get scared about going to school? Is it hard for you to control or stop your worrying? Are there specific things, places, or situations that make you feel very anxious or afraid? Have you ever felt suddenly frightened, nervous, or anxious for no reason at all? If so, can you tell me about that?*

If yes, ask: *Do these experiences ever cause you significant trouble with your friends or family, at school, or in another setting?*

- If a specific phobia is elicited, proceed to specific phobia disorder criteria.
- If no, first proceed to panic disorder criteria. Then proceed to generalized anxiety disorder criteria.

1. Specific Phobia [F40.2xx, 197–202]

   a. Inclusion: Requires that for at least 6 months, a person has experienced marked fear or anxiety as characterized by the following <u>three</u> symptoms.

      i. Specific fear: *Do you fear a specific object or situation such as flying, heights, animals, or something else so much that being exposed to it makes you feel immediately afraid or anxious? What is it?*

      ii. Fear or anxiety provoked by exposure: *When you encounter this, do you experience an immediate sense of fear or anxiety, cry, throw tantrums, or hold on to a parent?*

      iii. Avoidance: *Do you find yourself taking steps to avoid this? What are they? When you have to encounter this, do you experience intense fear or anxiety, cry, throw tantrums, or hold on to a parent?*

b. Exclusion: The fear, anxiety, and avoidance are not restricted to objects or situations related to obsessions, reminders of traumatic events, separation from home or attachment figures, or social situations.

c. Modifiers

    i. Specifiers

- Animal
- Natural environment
- Blood-injection-injury
- Situational
- Other

d. Alternatives

    i. If a young person reports developmentally inappropriate and excessive distress when separated from home or a major attachment figure or expresses persistent worry that his major attachment figure will be harmed or will die, which results in reluctance or refusal to be separated from home or a major attachment figure, consider separation anxiety disorder [F93.0, 190–195]. The onset of this disorder is before age 18. The minimum duration of symptoms necessary to meet the diagnostic criteria is 4 weeks for children and adolescents.

    ii. If a young person consistently fails to speak in specific social situations for at least 1 month, interfering with educational or occupational achievement, consider selective mutism [F94.0, 195–197]. If the disturbance is due to a lack of knowledge of, or comfort with, the spoken language, do not use this diagnosis. If the disturbance is better explained by a communication disorder, autism spectrum disorder, or psychotic disorder, do not use this diagnosis.

    iii. If a young person reports at least 6 months of marked and disproportionate fear or anxiety about situations such as public transportation, open spaces, being in shops or theaters, standing in line or being in a crowd, or being outside of the home alone, and if these fears cause him or her to actively avoid these situations, consider agoraphobia [F40.00, 217–221].

iv. If a young person reports at least 6 months of marked fear or anxiety about, or avoidance of, social situations in which he fears that other people will observe or scrutinize him or her out of proportion to the actual threat posed by these social situations, these social situations provoke fear or anxiety, and these situations are either avoided or endured, consider social anxiety disorder (social phobia) [F40.10, 202–208]. In children, the anxiety must occur with peers, not just with adults. Children may express fear or anxiety by crying, tantrums, freezing, clinging, shrinking, or failing to speak in social situations.

2. Panic Disorder [F41.0, 208–214]

a. Inclusion: Requires recurrent panic attacks, as characterized by at least <u>four</u> of the following symptoms:

i. Palpitations, pounding heart, or accelerated heart rate: *When you experience these sudden surges of intense fear or discomfort, does your heart race or pound?*

ii. Sweating: *During these events, do you find yourself sweating more than usual?*

iii. Trembling or shaking: *During these events, do you shake or develop a tremor?*

iv. Sensations of shortness of breath or smothering: *During these events, do you feel like you are being smothered or cannot catch your breath?*

v. Feelings of choking: *During these events, do you feel as though you are choking, as if something is blocking your throat?*

vi. Chest pain or discomfort: *During these events, do you feel intense pain or discomfort in your chest?*

vii. Nausea or abdominal distress: *During these events, do you feel sick to your stomach or like you need to vomit?*

viii. Feeling dizzy, unsteady, light-headed, or faint: *During these events, do you feel dizzy, light-headed, or like you may faint?*

ix. Chills or heat sensations: *During these events, do you feel very cold and shiver, or do you feel intensely hot?*

x. Paresthesias: *During these events, do you feel numbness or tingling?*

xi. Derealization or depersonalization: *During these events, do you feel as if people or places that are familiar to you are unreal or that you are so detached from your body that it is like you are standing outside your body or watching yourself?*

    xii. Fear of losing control: *During these events, do you fear you may be losing control or even "going crazy?"*

   xiii. Fear of dying: *During these events, do you fear you may be dying?*

  b. Inclusion: At least one panic attack is followed by at least 1 month of at least <u>one</u> of the following symptoms:

    i. Persistent worry about consequences: *Are you persistently concerned or worried about additional panic attacks? Are you persistently concerned or worried that these attacks mean you are having a heart attack, losing control, or "going crazy"?*

    ii. Maladaptive changes to avoid attacks: *Have you made significant changes in your behavior, such as avoiding unfamiliar situations or exercise, in order to avoid attacks?*

  c. Exclusion: If the disturbance is better explained by another mental disorder or is attributable to the physiological effects of a substance/medication or another medical condition, do not use this diagnosis.

  d. Alternatives

    i. If a young person reports panic attacks as described above but neither experiences persistent worry about consequences nor makes maladaptive changes to avoid attacks, consider using the panic attack specifier (DSM-5, pp. 214–217). The panic attack specifier can be used with other anxiety disorders, as well as with depressive, traumatic, and substance use disorders.

3. Generalized Anxiety Disorder [F41.1, 222–226]

  a. Inclusion: Requires excessive anxiety and worry that is difficult to control, occurring more days than not for at least 6 months, about a number of events or activities (such as school performance), associated with at least <u>three</u> of the following symptoms.

    i. Restlessness: *When you think about events or activities that make you anxious or worried, do you feel restless, on edge, or "keyed up?"*

    ii. Easily fatigued: *Do you find that you often tire or fatigue easily?*

iii. Difficulty concentrating: *When you are anxious or worried, do you often find it hard to concentrate or find that your mind goes blank?*

iv. Irritability: *When you are anxious or worried, do you often feel irritable or easily annoyed?*

v. Muscle tension: *When you get anxious or worried, do you often experience muscle tightness or tension?*

vi. Sleep disturbance: *Do you find it difficult to fall asleep or stay asleep or experience restless and unsatisfying sleep?*

b. Exclusion: If the anxiety and worry are better explained by another mental disorder or are attributable to the physiological effects of a substance/medication or another medical condition, do not use this diagnosis.

c. Alternatives

i. If a substance directly causes the episode, including a medication prescribed to treat a mental disorder, consider a substance/medication-induced anxiety disorder [F1x.x8x, 226–230].

ii. If another medical condition directly causes the anxiety and worry, consider an anxiety disorder due to another medical condition [F06.4, 230–232].

iii. If a young person experiences symptoms characteristic of an anxiety disorder that cause clinically significant distress or functional impairment without meeting full criteria for another anxiety disorder, consider unspecified anxiety disorder [F41.9, 233]. If you wish to communicate the specific reason a young person's symptoms do not meet the criteria for a specific anxiety disorder, consider other specified anxiety disorder [F41.8, 233]. Examples include generalized anxiety not occurring more days than not and *ataque de nervios* (attack of nerves).

Obsessive-Compulsive and Related Disorders

DSM-5 pp. 235–264

Screening question: *Do you ever get unwanted thoughts, urges, or pictures stuck in your mind and repeating that you cannot get rid of? Is there anything you feel you have to check, clean, or organize over and over again in order to feel OK?*

If yes, ask: *Do these experiences or behaviors ever cause you significant trouble with your friends or family, at school, or in another setting?*

- If yes, proceed to obsessive-compulsive disorder criteria.
- If no, proceed to the body-focused repetitive behavior screening question, which follows the obsessive-compulsive disorder section.

1. Obsessive-Compulsive Disorder [F42, 237–242]

   a. Inclusion: Requires the presence of obsessive thoughts, compulsive behaviors, or both, as manifested by the following symptoms.

      i. Obsessive thoughts: *When you experience these unwanted images, thoughts, or urges, do they make you anxious or distressed? Do you have to work hard to ignore or suppress these kinds of thoughts?*

      ii. Compulsive behaviors: *Some people try to reverse intrusive ideas by repeatedly performing some kind of action such as hand washing or lock checking or by a mental act such as counting, praying, or silently repeating words. Do you do something like that? Do you think that doing so will reduce your distress or prevent something from occurring?*

   b. Inclusion: The obsessions or compulsions are time-consuming (e.g., take more than 1 hour per day) or cause clinically significant distress or impairment.

   c. Exclusions

      i. If the obsessions or compulsions are better explained by another mental disorder, do not use this diagnosis.

      ii. If the obsessive-compulsive symptoms are attributable to the physiological effects of a substance, do not use this diagnosis.

      iii. If a young person reports that his intrusive images, thoughts, or urges are pleasurable, he does not meet the criteria for an obsessive-compulsive disorder.

   d. Modifiers

      i. Specifiers

         - Insight

            - With good or fair insight: Use if a person recognizes that his beliefs are definitely or probably untrue.

- With poor insight: Use if a person thinks his beliefs are probably true.
- With absent insight/delusional beliefs: Use if a person is completely convinced his beliefs are true.

ii. Tic-related: Use if a young person meets criteria for a current or lifetime chronic tic disorder.

e. Alternatives

i. If a person reports intrusive images, thoughts, or urges centered on his body image, consider body dysmorphic disorder [F45.22, 242–247]. The criteria include preoccupation with perceived defects in physical appearance beyond concern about weight or body fat in a person with an eating disorder, repetitive behaviors or mental acts in response to concern about appearance, and clinically significant distress or impairments because of the preoccupation.

ii. If a person reports persistent difficulty in parting with possessions regardless of their value, consider hoarding disorder [F42, 247–251]. The criteria include strong urges to save items, distress associated with discarding items, and the accumulation of a large number of possessions that clutter the home or workplace to the extent that it can no longer be used for its intended function.

iii. If a substance directly causes the condition, including a substance prescribed to treat depression, consider substance/medication-induced obsessive-compulsive and related disorder [F1x.x88, 257–260].

iv. If another medical condition directly causes the episode, consider obsessive-compulsive and related disorder due to another medical condition [F06.8, 260–263].

v. If a young person reports intrusive images, thoughts, or urges centered on more real-world concerns, consider an anxiety disorder.

vi. If a person experiences symptoms characteristic of an obsessive-compulsive and related disorder that cause clinically significant distress or functional impairment without meeting full criteria for another obsessive-compulsive and related disorder, consider unspecified obsessive-compulsive and related disorder [F42, 264]. If you wish to communicate the specific reason a person's symptoms do not meet the criteria for a specific obsessive-compulsive and related disorder, consider other specified obsessive-compulsive and related disorder [F42, 263–264]. Examples include body-focused repetitive behavior disorder, obsessional jealousy, and *koro*.

2. Body-Focused Repetitive Behaviors

   a. Inclusion: DSM-5 includes two conditions, trichotillomania (hair-pulling disorder) [F63.3, 251–254] and excoriation (skin-picking) disorder [L98.1, 254–257], with identically structured criteria. Either diagnosis requires the presence of <u>all three</u> of the following symptoms, plus distress or impairment caused by the symptoms.

      i. Behavior: *Do you frequently pull your hair or pick at your skin so much that it has caused hair loss or skin lesions?*

      ii. Repeated attempts to change: *Have you repeatedly tried to decrease or stop this behavior?*

      iii. Impairment: *Does this behavior cause you to feel ashamed or out of control? Do you avoid school or social settings because of these behaviors?*

   b. Exclusion

      i. If the behavior is associated with another medical condition or mental disorder or is the result of substance use, the behavior should be diagnostically accounted for with those conditions, and you should not diagnose either trichotillomania or excoriation disorder.

Trauma- and Stressor-Related Disorders

DSM-5 pp. 265–290

Screening question: *What is the worst thing that has ever happened to you? Has anyone ever touched you in a way did not want? Have you ever experienced or witnessed an event in which you were seriously injured or your life was in danger or you thought you were going to be seriously injured or endangered?*

If yes, ask: *Do you think about or reexperience these events? Does thinking about these experiences ever cause significant trouble with your friends or family, at school, or in another setting?*

- If yes, proceed to posttraumatic stress disorder criteria.
- If a child says no but his family or caregivers report disturbances in his primary attachments, proceed to reactive attachment disorder criteria.

1. Posttraumatic Stress Disorder [F43.10, 271–280]

   a. Inclusion: Requires exposure to actual or threatened death, serious injury, or sexual violation. The exposure can be firsthand or witnessed. In a child 6 years or younger, the traumatic exposure can be learning of the trauma experienced by a parent or caregiver. In a person older than 6 years, the traumatic exposure also can be learning of the trauma experienced by a parent or caregiver, but the experienced trauma must be violent or accidental. In addition, a person must experience at least <u>one</u> of the following intrusion symptoms for at least 1 month after the traumatic experience.

      i. Memories: *After that experience, did you ever experience intrusive memories of the experience when you did not want to think about it?* For young children, repetitive reenactment through play qualifies: *Do you repeatedly reenact that experience with your toys or dolls when playing?*

      ii. Dreams: *Did you have recurrent, distressing dreams related to the experience?* For young children, frightening dreams without recognizable content qualifies: *Do you frequently have very frightening dreams that you cannot recall or describe?*

      iii. Flashbacks: *After that experience, did you ever feel as if it were happening to you again, like in a flashback?* For young children, this may be observed in their play.

      iv. Exposure distress: *When you are around people, places, and objects that remind you of that experience, do you feel intense or prolonged distress?*

      v. Physiological reactions: *When you are around people, places, or objects that remind you of that experience, do you have distressing physical responses?*

b. Inclusion: In addition, a young person older than 6 years must experience at least <u>one</u> of the following avoidance symptoms after the traumatic experience. For a child 6 years or younger, no negative mood symptoms need be experienced if at least <u>one</u> negative mood symptom (see item c below) is present.

  i. Internal reminders: *Do you work hard to avoid thoughts, feelings, or physical sensations that bring up memories of this experience?*

  ii. External reminders: *Do you work hard to avoid people, places, and objects that bring up memories of this experience?*

c. Inclusion: In addition, a young person older than 6 years must experience at least <u>two</u> of the following negative symptoms. For a child 6 years or younger, no negative mood symptoms need be experienced if at least <u>one</u> avoidance symptom (see item b above) is present.

  i. Impaired memory: *Do you have trouble remembering important parts of the experience?*

  ii. Negative self-image: *Do you frequently think negative thoughts about yourself, other people, or the world?*

  iii. Blame: *Do you frequently blame yourself or others for your experience, even when you know that you or they were not responsible?*

  iv. Negative emotional state: *Do you stay down, angry, ashamed, or fearful most of the time?*

  v. Decreased participation: *Are you much less interested in activities in which you used to participate?*

  vi. Detachment: *Do you feel detached or estranged from the people in your life because of this experience?*

  vii. Inability to experience positive emotion: *Do you find that you cannot feel happy, loved, or satisfied? Do you feel numb or as if you cannot love?*

d. Inclusion: In addition, a young person must experience at least <u>two</u> of the following arousal behaviors.

  i. Irritable or aggressive: *Do you often act very grumpy or get aggressive?*

  ii. Reckless: *Do you often act reckless or self-destructive?*

  iii. Hypervigilance: *Are you always on edge or keyed up?*

  iv. Exaggerated startle: *Do you startle easily?*

> v. Impaired concentration: *Do you often have trouble concentrating on a task or problem?*
> vi. Sleep disturbance: *Do you often have difficulty falling asleep or staying asleep, or do you often wake up without feeling rested?*

e. Exclusions

> i. If the witnessing of traumatic events includes events witnessed only in electronic media, television, movies, or pictures, do not use this diagnosis.
> ii. If the episode is directly caused by the use of a substance or by another medical condition, do not use this diagnosis.

f. Modifiers

> i. Subtypes
>
> • With dissociative symptoms: depersonalization
> • With dissociative symptoms: derealization
>
> ii. Specifiers
>
> • With delayed expression: Use if a person does not meet all the diagnostic criteria until at least 6 months after the traumatic experience.

g. Alternatives

> i. If the episode lasts less than 1 month and the experience occurred within the past month and the young person experiences at least <u>nine</u> of the posttraumatic symptoms described earlier, consider acute stress disorder [F43.0, 280–286].
> ii. If the episode began within 3 months of the experience and a young person does not meet the symptomatic and behavioral criteria for posttraumatic stress disorder, consider an adjustment disorder [F43.2x, 286–289]. The criteria include marked distress disproportionate to an acute stressor, either traumatic or nontraumatic, and significant impairment in function.
> iii. If a young person experiences symptoms characteristic of a trauma- and stressor-related disorder that cause clinically significant distress or functional impairment without meeting full criteria for one of the named disorders, consider unspecified trauma- and stressor-related disorder [F43.9, 290]. If you wish to communicate the specific rea-

son a young person's symptoms do not meet the criteria for a specific disorder, consider other specified trauma- and stressor-related disorder [F43.8, 289]. Examples include adjustment-like disorders with delayed onset of symptoms that occur more than 3 months after the stressor.

2. Reactive Attachment Disorder [F94.1, 265–268]

This section contains questions phrased for interviewing an older child with an ability to self-reflect. For younger children or those with limited cognitive functioning, rephrase these questions to interview the child's caregiver instead.

a. Inclusion: Requires that a child experience pathogenic care, before age 5 years, that results in <u>both</u> of the following behaviors.

   i. Rare or minimal comfort seeking: *When you are feeling really angry, upset, or sad, do you avoid comfort or consolation from other people?*

   ii. Rare or minimal response to comfort: *When you are feeling really angry, upset, or sad, and somebody says or does something nice for you, does it make you feel a little better?*

b. Inclusion: Requires the persistent experience of at least <u>two</u> of the following states.

   i. Relative lack of social and emotional responsiveness to others: *When you interact with other people, do you usually have very little feeling or emotion?*

   ii. Limited positive affect: *Do you usually find it hard to be excited or to feel good or cheerful?*

   iii. Episodes of unexplained irritability, sadness, or fearfulness, which are evident during nonthreatening interactions with caregivers: *Do you often have episodes where you become irritable, sad, or afraid with an adult caregiver who does not pose a threat to you?*

c. Inclusion: Requires the persistent experience of at least <u>one</u> of the following states that should be assessed in the social history.

   i. Social neglect or deprivation in the form of persistent lack of having basic emotional needs for comfort, stimulation, and affection met.

   ii. Repeated changes of primary caregivers that limit opportunities to form stable attachments.

  iii. Rearing in unusual settings that severely limit opportunities to form selective attachments.

 d. Exclusions

  i. If a child does not have a developmental age of at least 9 months, do not use this diagnosis.

  ii. If a child meets criteria for autism spectrum disorder, do not use this diagnosis.

 e. Modifier

  i. Specifier

   • Persistent: Use when the disorder is present for more than 12 months.

  ii. Severity: Specified severe when a child meets all symptoms of the disorder, with each symptom manifesting in relatively high levels.

 f. Alternative: If a young child who has experienced extremes of insufficient care shows profoundly disturbed externalizing behavior, consider disinhibited social engagement disorder [F94.2, 268–270]. The criteria include at least <u>two</u> of the following symptoms: reduced reticence with unfamiliar adults, overly familiar verbal or physical behavior, diminished checking back with adult caregiver after venturing away, and a willingness to go off with an unfamiliar adult with reduced hesitation.

Dissociative Disorders

DSM-5 pp. 291–307

Screening question: *Everyone has trouble remembering things sometimes, but do you ever lose time, forget important details about yourself, or find evidence that you took part in events that you cannot recall? Do you ever feel as if people or places that are familiar to you are unreal or that you are so detached from your body that it is like you are standing outside your body or watching yourself?*

 If yes, ask: *Did these experiences ever cause you significant trouble with your friends or family, at school, or in another setting?*

• If amnesia predominates, proceed to dissociative amnesia criteria.

• If depersonalization or derealization predominates, proceed to depersonalization/derealization disorder criteria.

1. Dissociative Amnesia [F44.0, 298–302]

   a. Inclusion: Requires the presence of inability to recall important autobiographical information beyond ordinary forgetting, most often manifested by at least <u>one</u> of the following symptoms.

      i. Localized or selective amnesia: *Do you find yourself unable to recall a really important event, especially events that were especially stressful or even traumatic?*

      ii. Generalized amnesia: *Do you find yourself unable to recall really important moments in your life history or details of your very identity?*

   b. Exclusions

      i. If the disturbance is better accounted for by dissociative identity disorder, posttraumatic stress disorder, acute stress disorder, or somatic symptom disorder, do not use this diagnosis.

      ii. If the disturbance is due to the physiological effects of a substance or a neurological or other medical condition, do not use this diagnosis.

   c. Modifiers

      i. Specifier

         • With dissociative fugue [F44.1, 298]: Use when a person engages in purposeful travel or bewildered wandering for which he has amnesia.

   d. Alternative: If a young person reports a disruption of identity, characterized by two or more distinct personality states or an experience of possession, that causes clinically significant distress and functional impairment, consider dissociative identity disorder [F44.81, 292–298]. The criteria include recurrent gaps in recall that are inconsistent with ordinary forgetting and dissociative experiences that are not a normal part of a broadly accepted cultural or religious practice and that are not attributable to the physiological effects of a substance or another medical condition.

2. Depersonalization/Derealization Disorder [F48.1, 302–306]

   a. Inclusion: Requires at least <u>one</u> of the following manifestations.

      i. Depersonalization: *Do you frequently have experiences of unreality or detachment—as if you are an outside ob-*

server of your mind, thoughts, feelings, sensations, body, or your whole self?

    ii. Derealization: *Do you frequently have experiences of unreality or detachment for your surroundings—that you often experience people or places as unreal, dream-like, foggy, lifeless, or visually distorted?*

b. Inclusion: Requires intact reality testing. *During these experiences, can you distinguish the experiences from actual events—what is occurring outside of you?*

c. Exclusions

    i. If the disturbance is due to the physiological effects of a substance or a neurological or other medical condition, do not use this diagnosis.

    ii. If depersonalization or derealization occurs exclusively as symptoms of or during the course of another mental disorder, do not use this diagnosis.

d. Alternative: If a young person is experiencing a disorder whose most prominent symptoms are amnestic but does not meet the criteria for a specific disorder, consider unspecified dissociative disorder [F44.9, 307]. If you wish to communicate the specific reason a young person's symptoms do not meet criteria for a specific disorder, consider other specified dissociative disorder [F44.89, 306–307]. Examples include subthreshold dissociative disturbances in identity and memory, chronic and recurrent syndromes of mixed dissociative symptoms, identity disturbances in individuals subjected to prolonged periods of intense coercive persuasion, acute reactions to stressful situations, acute psychotic states intermixed with dissociative symptoms in a person who does not meet criteria for delirium or a psychotic disorder, and dissociative trance.

Somatic Symptom and Related Disorders

DSM-5 pp. 309–327

Screening question: *Do you worry about your physical health more than most young people? Do you get sick more often than most young people?*

    If yes, ask: *Do these experiences significantly affect your daily life at home or in school?*

If yes, ask: *Which is worse for you, worrying about the symptoms you experience or worrying about your health and the possibility that you are sick?*

- If worry about symptoms predominates, proceed to somatic symptom disorder criteria.
- If worry about being ill or sick predominates, proceed to illness anxiety disorder criteria.

1. Somatic Symptom Disorder [F45.1, 311–315]

    a. Inclusion: Requires at least <u>one</u> somatic symptom that is distressing. *Do you experience symptoms that cause you to feel anxious or distressed? Do these symptoms significantly disrupt your daily life?*

    b. Inclusion: Requires at least <u>one</u> of the following thoughts, feelings, or behaviors, for at least 6 months.

        i. Disproportionate thoughts: *How serious are your health concerns, and do you think about them often?*

        ii. Persistently high level of anxiety: *Do you persistently feel a high level of anxiety or worry about your health concerns?*

        iii. Excessive investment: *Do you find yourself investing a lot more time and energy into your health concerns than you would like to?*

    c. Modifiers

        i. Specifiers

            - With predominant pain
            - Persistent

        ii. Severity

            - Mild: One of the additional symptoms specified in (b) above.
            - Moderate: Two or more of the additional symptoms specified in (b) above.
            - Severe: Two or more of the additional symptoms specified in (b) above plus multiple somatic complaints (or one very severe somatic symptom)

    d. Alternatives

        i. If a young person is focused on the loss of bodily function rather than on the distress a particular symptom causes, consider conversion disorder (functional neurological symptom disorder) [F44.x, 318–321]. The criteria for this disorder include symptoms or deficits affecting voluntary motor or sensory function, clinical evidence that these symptoms or deficits are inconsistent with a recognized medical or neurological disease, and significant impairment in social or occupational functioning.

ii. If a young person has a documented medical condition, but behavioral or psychological factors adversely affect the course of his medical condition by delaying recovery, decreasing adherence, significantly increasing health risks, or influencing the underlying pathophysiology, consider psychological factors affecting other medical conditions [F54, 322–324].

iii. If a young person falsifies physical or psychological signs or symptoms or induces injury or disease to deceptively present himself or herself to others as ill, impaired, or injured, consider factitious disorder imposed on self [F68.10, 324–326]. If a young person exhibits these behaviors in pursuit of obvious external rewards, as in malingering, do not use this diagnosis. If a young person's symptoms are better accounted for by another mental disorder, such as a psychotic disorder, do not use this diagnosis.

iv. If a person falsifies physical or psychological signs or symptoms or induces injury or disease to deceptively present someone else to others as ill, impaired, or injured, consider factitious disorder imposed on another [F68.10, 325–326]. The diagnosis is assigned to the perpetrator rather than the victim. If the perpetrator exhibits these behaviors in pursuit of obvious external rewards, as in malingering, do not use this diagnosis. If the perpetrator's behavior is better accounted for by another mental disorder, such as a psychotic disorder, do not use this diagnosis.

2. Illness Anxiety Disorder [F45.21, 315–318]

a. Inclusion: Requires all of the following symptoms for at least 6 months and the absence of somatic symptoms.

i. Preoccupation: *Do you find yourself unable to stop thinking about having or acquiring a serious illness?*
ii. Anxiety: *Do you feel a high level of anxiety or worry about having or acquiring a serious illness?*
iii. Associated behaviors: *Have these worries affected your behavior? Some people find themselves frequently checking their body for signs of illness; reading about illness all the time; or avoiding persons, places, or objects to ward off illness. Do you find yourself doing any of those things or things like that?*

b. Exclusion: If a person's symptoms are better explained by another mental disorder, do not use this diagnosis.
c. Modifiers

i. Subtypes

• Care-seeking type
• Care-avoidant type

ii. Course

• Transient

d. Alternatives: If a young person endorses symptoms characteristic of a somatic symptom and related disorder that cause clinically significant distress or impairment without meeting the full criteria for a specific disorder, consider unspecified somatic symptom and related disorder [F45.9, 327]. If you wish to communicate the specific reason a young person's symptoms do not meet criteria for a specific disorder, consider other specified somatic symptom and related disorder [F45.8, 327]. Examples include brief somatic symptom disorder, brief illness anxiety disorder, illness anxiety disorder without excessive health-related behaviors, and pseudocyesis.

Feeding and Eating Disorders

DSM-5 pp. 329–354

Screening question: *What do you think of your appearance? Do you ever restrict or avoid particular foods so much that it negatively affects your health or weight?*

If yes, ask: *When you consider yourself, is the shape or weight of your body one of the most important things about you?*

- If yes, proceed to anorexia nervosa criteria.
- If no, proceed to avoidant/restrictive food intake disorder criteria.

1. Anorexia Nervosa [F50.0x, 338–345]

    a. Inclusion: Requires the presence of all <u>three</u> of the following features.

        i. Energy restriction leading to significantly low body weight adjusted for age, developmental trajectory, physical health, and sex: *Have you limited the food you eat to achieve a low body weight? What was the least you ever weighed? What do you weigh now?*

        ii. Fear of weight gain or behavior interfering with weight gain: *Do you have an intense fear of gaining weight or becoming fat? Has there ever been a time when you were already at a low weight and still did things to interfere with gaining weight?*

        iii. Disturbance in self-perceived weight or shape: *How do you experience the weight and shape of your body? How do you think having a significantly low body weight will affect your physical health?*

    b. Modifiers

        i. Subtypes

            - Restricting type [F50.01, 339]: Use when a young person reports no recurrent episodes of binge eating or purging in the last 3 months.
            - Binge-eating/purging type [F50.02, 339]: Use when a young person reports recurrent episodes of binge eating or purging in the last 3 months.

        ii. Specifiers

            - In partial remission
            - In full remission

        iii. Severity

            - Mild: Age- and gender-matched percentiles equivalent to adult body mass index (BMI) $\geq 17 \text{ kg/m}^2$
            - Moderate: Age- and gender-matched percentiles equivalent to adult BMI $16–16.99 \text{ kg/m}^2$
            - Severe: Age- and gender-matched percentiles equivalent to adult BMI $15–15.99 \text{ kg/m}^2$

- Extreme: Age- and gender-matched percentiles equivalent to adult BMI < 15 kg/m^2

c. Alternatives

   i. If a young person reports recurrent binge eating, recurrent inappropriate compensatory behaviors to prevent weight gain (e.g., misuse of laxatives or other medications, self-induced vomiting, excessive exercise), and self-image unduly influenced by the shape or weight of his body, consider bulimia nervosa [F50.2, 345–350]. The diagnosis requires that binge eating and compensatory behaviors both occur, on average, at least once a week for 3 months. If binge eating and compensating behaviors occur only during episodes of anorexia nervosa, the diagnosis should not be given.

2. Avoidant/Restrictive Food Intake Disorder [F50.8, 334–338]

   a. Inclusion: Requires significant disturbance in eating or feeding manifested by persistent failure to meet appropriate nutritional and/or energy needs associated with at least <u>one</u> of the following sequelae.

      i. Faltering growth or significant weight loss: *Do you avoid certain foods or restrict what you eat to the extent that you have not grown at the expected rate or have experienced a significant weight loss?*

      ii. Significant nutritional deficiency: *Do you avoid or restrict food to the extent that it has negatively affected your health, as in experiencing a significant nutritional deficiency?*

      iii. Dependence on enteral feeding or oral supplements: *Have you avoided or restricted food to the extent that you depend on tube feedings or oral supplements to maintain nutrition?*

      iv. Marked interference with psychosocial functioning: *Can you eat with other people or participate in social activities when food is present? Has avoiding or restricting food impaired your ability to participate in your usual social activities or made it hard to form or sustain relationships?*

   b. Exclusions

      i. If the eating disturbance is better explained by lack of available food, by an associated culturally sanctioned practice, or by eating practices related to a disturbance in body image, do not use this diagnosis.

    ii. If the eating disturbance is due to another medical condition or is better explained by another mental disorder, do not use this diagnosis.

c. Alternatives

    i. If a young person persistently eats nonfood substances over a period of at least 1 month, consider pica [F98.3, 329–331]. The eating of nonnutritive, nonfood substances must be inappropriate to his developmental stage and must not be part of a culturally supported or socially normative practice.

    ii. If a young person repeatedly regurgitates food over a period of at least 1 month, consider rumination disorder [F98.21, 332–333]. If the regurgitation occurs as the result of an associated gastrointestinal or other medical condition or occurs exclusively during the course of anorexia nervosa, bulimia nervosa, binge-eating disorder, or avoidant/restrictive food intake disorder, do not use this diagnosis.

    iii. If a young person has an atypical, mixed, or subthreshold disturbance in his eating and feeding, or if you lack sufficient information to make a more specific diagnosis, consider unspecified feeding or eating disorder [F50.9, 354]. DSM-5 also allows the use of this category for specific syndromes that are not formally included, such as purging disorder. If you wish to communicate the specific reason a young person's symptoms do not meet criteria for a specific disorder, consider other specified feeding or eating disorder [F50.8, 353–354]. Examples include atypical anorexia nervosa, binge-eating disorder, and purging disorder.

Elimination Disorders

DSM-5 pp. 355–360

Screening question: *Have you repeatedly passed urine or feces onto your clothing, your bed, the floor, or another inappropriate place?*

- If passing urine, proceed to enuresis criteria.
- If passing feces, proceed to encopresis criteria.

1. Enuresis [F98.0, 355–357]

   a. Inclusion

      i. Intentional or involuntary voiding of urine: *On average, have you been urinating like this at least two times a week?*

      ii. Duration: *Has this urinating occurred for at least 3 months in a row?*

   b. Exclusions

      i. If a child is younger than 5 years, or the equivalent developmental age, do not use this diagnosis.

      ii. If the behavior is due to the physiological effects of a substance or another medical condition through a mechanism other than constipation, do not use this diagnosis.

   c. Modifiers

      i. Nocturnal only

      ii. Diurnal only

      iii. Nocturnal and diurnal

   d. Alternatives

      i. If a young person experiences symptoms characteristic of an elimination disorder that cause clinically significant distress or impairment without meeting the full criteria for an elimination disorder, consider unspecified elimination disorder with urinary symptoms [R32, 360]. If you wish to communicate the specific reason that full criteria are not met, consider other specified elimination disorder with urinary symptoms [N39.498, 359].

2. Encopresis [F98.1, 357–359]

   a. Inclusion

      i. Intentional or involuntary voiding of feces: *On average, have you been defecating like this at least once a month?*

      ii. Duration: *Has this defecating occurred for at least 3 months in a row?*

   b. Exclusions

      i. If a child is younger than 4 years, or the equivalent developmental age, do not use this diagnosis.

      ii. If the behavior is due to the physiological effects of a substance or another medical condition through a mechanism other than constipation, do not use this diagnosis.

c. Modifiers

   i. With constipation and overflow incontinence

   ii. Without constipation and overflow incontinence

d. Alternatives

   i. If a young person experiences symptoms characteristic of an elimination disorder that cause clinically significant distress or impairment without meeting the full criteria for an elimination disorder, consider unspecified elimination disorder with fecal symptoms [R15.9, 360]. If you wish to communicate the specific reason that full criteria are not met, consider other specified elimination disorder with fecal symptoms [R15.9, 359].

Sleep-Wake Disorders

DSM-5 pp. 361–422

Screening question: *Is your sleep often inadequate or of poor quality? Alternatively, do you often experience excessive sleepiness? Have you, or someone else, noticed any unusual behaviors while you sleep? Have you, or someone else, noticed that you stop breathing or gasp for air while sleeping?*

- If dissatisfaction with sleep quantity or quality predominates, proceed to insomnia disorder criteria.
- If excessive sleep predominates, proceed to hypersomnolence disorder criteria.
- If an irrepressible need to sleep or sudden lapses into sleep predominate, proceed to narcolepsy criteria.
- If unusual sleep behaviors (parasomnias) predominate, proceed to restless legs syndrome criteria.
- If sleep-breathing problems predominate, proceed to obstructive sleep apnea hypopnea criteria.

1. Insomnia Disorder [F51.01, 362–368]

   a. Inclusion: Requires dissatisfaction with sleep quantity or quality, at least 3 nights per week, for at least 3 months, as manifested by at least <u>one</u> of the following symptoms.

i. Difficulty initiating sleep: *Do you often have trouble getting to sleep without the help of a parent or someone else?*

ii. Difficulty maintaining sleep: *If you wake up when you wanted to be asleep, do you need the help of a parent or someone else to get back to sleep?*

iii. Early-morning awakening: *Do you often wake up earlier than you intended and find yourself unable to return to sleep?*

b. Exclusions

   i. If a young person does not have adequate opportunity for sleep, do not use this diagnosis.

   ii. If a young person's insomnia is better explained by another sleep-wake disorder, another mental disorder, or another medical condition, do not use this diagnosis.

   iii. If the physiological effects of a substance cause a young person's insomnia, do not use this diagnosis.

c. Modifiers

   i. Specifiers

   • With non–sleep disorder mental comorbidity, including substance use disorders
   • With other medical comorbidity
   • With other sleep disorder

   ii. Course

   • Episodic: symptoms last between 1 and 3 months
   • Persistent: symptoms last 3 months or longer
   • Recurrent: At least two episodes within 1 year

d. Alternatives

   i. If a young person experiences a persistent or recurrent pattern of sleep disruption leading to excessive sleepiness, insomnia, or both, and this disruption is primarily due to an alteration of the circadian system or to a misalignment between the endogenous circadian rhythm and the sleep-wake schedule required by a person's physical environment or social or professional schedule, consider a circadian rhythm sleep-wake disorder [G47.2x, 390–398]. The sleep disturbance must cause clinically significant distress or functional impairment.

Subtypes include delayed sleep phase type, advanced sleep phase type, and irregular sleep-wake type.

ii. If substance use, intoxication, or withdrawal is etiologically related to insomnia that causes significant distress or impairment, consider substance/medication-induced sleep disorder, insomnia type [F1x.x92, 413–420]. If the insomnia is better accounted for by delirium, a non-substance-induced sleep disorder, or the sleep symptoms usually associated with an intoxication or withdrawal syndrome, this diagnosis should not be used.

iii. If a young person experiences symptoms characteristic of an insomnia disorder that cause clinically significant distress or impairment without meeting criteria for a disorder, consider unspecified insomnia disorder [G47.00, 420]. If you wish to communicate the specific reason that full criteria are not met, consider other specified insomnia disorder [G47.09, 420]. Examples include brief insomnia disorder and insomnia restricted to nonrestorative sleep.

2. Hypersomnolence Disorder [F51.11, 368–372]

a. Inclusion: Requires excessive sleepiness at least three times per week for at least 3 months, despite a main sleep period lasting at least 7 hours, that causes significant distress or functional impairment. The hypersomnolence is manifested by at least <u>one</u> of the following symptoms.

i. Recurrent periods of sleep: *Do you often have several periods of sleep within the same day?*

ii. Prolonged nonrestorative sleep episode: *When you sleep for at least 9 hours, do you still wake up without feeling refreshed or restored?*

iii. Sleep inertia: *Do you often have difficulty being fully awake? After an awakening, do you often feel groggy or notice that you have trouble engaging in tasks or activities that would otherwise be simple for you?*

b. Exclusion: If the hypersomnia occurs exclusively during the course of another sleep disorder, is better accounted for by another sleep disorder, or is attributable to the physiological effects of a substance, do not use this diagnosis.

c. Modifiers

   i. Specifiers

- With mental disorder, including substance use disorders
- With medical condition
- With another sleep disorder

   ii. Course

- Acute: duration of less than 1 month
- Subacute: duration of 1–3 months
- Persistent: duration of more than 3 months

   iii. Severity

- Mild: difficulty maintaining daytime alertness 1–2 days/week
- Moderate: difficulty maintaining daytime alertness 3–4 days/week
- Severe: difficulty maintaining daytime alertness 5–7 days/week

d. Alternative: If substance use, intoxication, or withdrawal is etiologically related to daytime sleepiness, consider substance/medication-induced sleep disorder, daytime sleepiness type [F1x.x92, 413–420]. If the disturbance is better accounted for by delirium, a non–substance-induced sleep disorder, or the sleep symptoms usually associated with an intoxication or withdrawal syndrome, this diagnosis should not be used.

3. Narcolepsy [G47.4xx, 372–378]

a. Inclusion: Requires periods of an irrepressible need to sleep or lapsing into sleep, at least three times per week over the past 3 months, along with at least <u>one</u> of the following.

   i. Episodes of cataplexy: *At least a few times a month, do you find that all of a sudden you grimace, open your mouth wide and thrust out your tongue, or lose muscle tone throughout your body?*

   ii. Hypocretin deficiency: Measured using cerebrospinal fluid hypocretin-1 (CSF-1) immunoreactivity values.

   iii. Nocturnal sleep polysomnography showing rapid eye movement (REM) sleep latency of 15 minutes or less or a multiple sleep latency test showing mean sleep latency of 8 minutes or less and two or more sleep-onset REM periods.

b. Modifiers

   i. Specifiers

   • Narcolepsy without cataplexy but with hypo-cretin deficiency: low CSF-1 levels and positive polysomnograpy/multiple sleep latency test but no cataplexy

   • Narcolepsy with cataplexy but without hypo-cretin deficiency: cataplexy and positive poly-somnograpy/multiple sleep latency test but normal CSF-1 levels

   • Autosomal dominant cerebellar ataxia, deafness, and narcolepsy: subtype caused by exon 21 DNA (cytosine-5)-methyltransferase-1 mutations and characterized by late-onset (age 30–40 years) narcolepsy (with low or intermediate CSF hypo-cretin-1 levels), deafness, cerebellar ataxia, and eventually dementia

   • Autosomal dominant narcolepsy, obesity, and type 2 diabetes: Narcolepsy, obesity, and type 2 diabetes and low CSF-1 levels associated with a mutation in the myelin oligodendrocyte gly-coprotein gene

   • Narcolepsy secondary to another medical con-dition: Narcolepsy developing secondary to medical conditions that cause infectious (e.g., Whipple's disease, sarcoidosis), traumatic, or tumoral destruction of hypocretin neurons

   ii. Severity

   • Mild: Infrequent cataplexy (less than once per week), need for naps only once or twice per day, and less disturbed nocturnal sleep

   • Moderate: Cataplexy once daily or every few days, disturbed nocturnal sleep, and need for multiple naps daily

   • Severe: Drug-resistant cataplexy with multiple attacks daily, nearly constant sleepiness, and disturbed nocturnal sleep (i.e., movements, in-somnia, and vivid dreaming)

4. Obstructive Sleep Apnea Hypopnea [G47.33, 378–383]

   a. Inclusion: Requires repeated episodes of upper air-way obstruction during sleep. There must be poly-somnographic evidence of at least five obstructive apneas or hypopneas per hour of sleep and <u>either</u> of the following symptoms.

   i. Nocturnal breathing disturbances: *Do you often disturb your parents, siblings, or anyone else with snoring, snorting, gasping for air, or breathing pauses during sleep?*

   ii. Daytime sleepiness, fatigue, or nonrestorative sleep that is not attributable to another medical condition or is not explained by psychiatric morbidity: *When you have an opportunity to get sleep, do you still wake up the next day feeling exhausted, sleepy, or fatigued?*

b. Inclusion: Alternatively, the diagnosis can be made by polysomnographic evidence of 15 or more obstructive apneas or hypopneas per hour of sleep regardless of accompanying symptoms.

c. Modifiers

   i. Severity

      • Mild: apnea hypopnea index less than 15
      • Moderate: apnea hypopnea index between 15 and 30
      • Severe: apnea hypopnea index greater than 30

d. Alternatives

   i. If a young person has five or more central apneas per hour of sleep during polysomnographic examination and this disturbance is not better accounted for by another current sleep disorder, consider central sleep apnea [G47.31, 383–386].

   ii. If a young person has episodes of shallow breathing associated with arterial oxygen desaturation and/or elevated carbon dioxide levels during polysomnographic examination and this disturbance is not better accounted for by another current sleep disorder, consider sleep-related hypoventilation [G47.3x, 387–390]. This disorder is most commonly associated with medical or neurological disorders, obesity, medication use, or substance use disorders.

5. Restless Legs Syndrome [G25.81, 410–413]

a. Inclusion: Requires an urge to move the legs, usually accompanied by or in response to uncomfortable and unpleasant sensations in the legs, at least three times per week for at least 3 months, as manifested by <u>all</u> of the following symptoms.

    i. Urge to move legs: *While you are asleep, do you often experience uncomfortable or unpleasant sensations in the legs? Do you often experience an urge to move your legs when you are otherwise inactive?*

    ii. Relieved with movement: *Are these symptoms partially or completely relieved by moving your legs?*

    iii. Nocturnal worsening: *What times of day do you most experience the urge to move your legs? Is it worse in the evening or at night, no matter what you have done during the day?*

b. Exclusions

    i. If a young person's restless legs are better explained by another mental disorder, another medical condition, or a behavioral condition, do not use this diagnosis.

    ii. If the physiological effects of a substance cause a young person's restless legs, do not use this diagnosis.

c. Alternatives

    i. If a young person experiences recurrent episodes of incomplete awakening from sleep in which he experiences an abrupt and terrifying awakening (sleep terror) or he rises from bed and walks about (sleepwalking), usually during the first third of the major sleep episode, consider non–rapid eye movement sleep arousal disorders [F51.x, 399–404]. When experiencing an episode, a person experiences little to no dream imagery. The young person experiences amnesia for the episode and is relatively unresponsive to efforts of other people.

    ii. If a young person repeatedly experiences extremely dysphoric and well-remembered dreams and rapidly becomes alert and oriented on awakening from these dysphoric dreams, consider nightmare disorder [F51.5, 404–407]. The dream disturbance, or the sleep disturbance produced by awakening from the nightmare, causes clinically significant distress or functional impairment. If the dysphoric dreams occur exclusively during another mental disorder or as the physiological effect of a substance or another medical condition, do not use this diagnosis.

iii. If a young person repeatedly experiences episodes of arousal from sleep associated with vocalization and/or complex motor behaviors sufficient to result in injury to himself or herself or his bed partner, consider rapid eye movement sleep behavior disorder [G47.52, 407–410]. These behaviors arise during REM sleep and typically occur more than 90 minutes after sleep onset. On awakening, the person is fully awake, alert, and oriented. The diagnosis requires either polysomnographic evidence of REM sleep disturbance or evidence that the behaviors are injurious, potentially injurious, or disruptive.

iv. If substance use, intoxication, or withdrawal is etiologically related to daytime sleepiness, consider substance/medication-induced sleep disorder, parasomnia type [F1x.x92, 413–420]. If the disturbance is better accounted for by delirium, a non-substance-induced sleep disorder, or the sleep symptoms usually associated with an intoxication or withdrawal syndrome, the diagnosis should not be given.

v. If a young person experiences symptoms characteristic of restless legs or another sleep disturbance that cause clinically significant distress or impairment without meeting criteria for a disorder, consider unspecified insomnia disorder [G47.00, 420]. If you wish to communicate the specific reason that full criteria are not met, consider other specified insomnia disorder G47.09, 420].

Gender Dysphoria

DSM-5 pp. 451–459

Screening question: *Are you really uncomfortable with your assigned gender?*

If yes, ask: *Has this discomfort lasted at least 6 months and gotten to the point where you really feel that your assigned gender is incongruent with your gender identity? Does this discomfort cause significant trouble with your friends or family, at school, or in another setting?*

- If a child says yes, proceed to gender dysphoria in children.
- If an adolescent says yes, proceed to gender dysphoria in adolescents.

1. Gender Dysphoria in Children [F64.2, 452–459]

   a. Inclusion: Requires at least <u>six</u> of the following manifestations (one of which must be a strong desire to be of the other gender) for at least 6 months' duration.

      i. Desire to be of other gender: *Have you experienced a strong desire to be of a gender other than your assigned gender? Do you insist that people treat you as a member of a gender other than your assigned gender?*

      ii. Cross-dressing: *Do you have a strong preference for clothes usually associated with a gender other than your assigned gender?*

      iii. Cross-gender fantasy: *When you play fantasy games, do you have a strong preference for cross-gender roles?*

      iv. Cross-gender play: *When you play, do you have a strong preference for toys or activities that most people associate with the other gender?*

      v. Cross-gender playmates: *Do you have a strong preference for friends of the other gender?*

      vi. Rejection of toys, games, and activities: *Do you strongly reject the toys, games, and activities typically associated with your assigned gender?*

      vii. Dislike of anatomy: *Do you have a strong dislike of your sexual anatomy?*

      viii. Desire to have other sex characteristics: *Have you experienced a strong desire for the primary or secondary sex characteristics that match your experience of gender?*

   b. Specifiers

      i. With a disorder of sex development

2. Gender Dysphoria in Adolescents [F64.1, 452–459]

   a. Inclusion: Requires at least <u>two</u> of the following manifestations for at least 6 months' duration.

      i. Incongruence: *Have you experienced a profound sense that your primary or secondary sex characteristics do not match your gender identity?*

      ii. Desire to change: *Have you experienced a profound desire to change your primary or secondary sex characteristics because they do not match your gender identity?*

    iii. Desire to have sexual characteristics of other gender: *Have you experienced a strong desire for the primary or secondary sex characteristics that match your experience of gender?*

    iv. Desire to be another gender: *Have you experienced a strong desire to be of a gender other than your assigned gender?*

    v. Desire to be treated as another gender: *Have you experienced a strong desire to be treated as a gender other than your assigned gender?*

    vi. Conviction that one has feelings of another gender: *Have you experienced a strong conviction that your typical feelings and reactions are those of the gender other than your assigned gender?*

b. Modifiers

  i. Specifiers

- With a disorder of sex development
- Posttransition: The individual has transitioned to full-time living in the desired gender (with or without legalization of gender change) and has undergone (or is preparing to have) at least one cross-sex medical procedure or treatment regimen.

c. Alternatives

  i. If a person experiences symptoms characteristic of gender dysphoria that cause clinically significant distress or impairment without meeting the full criteria for gender dysphoria, consider unspecified gender dysphoria [F64.9, 459]. If you wish to communicate the specific reason that a person's symptoms do not meet full criteria, consider other specified gender dysphoria [F64.8, 459].

Disruptive, Impulse-Control, and Conduct Disorders

DSM-5 pp. 461–480

Screening question: *Do you often have times when you become so upset that you make or even act on verbal or physical threats to hurt other people, animals, or property? Have you ever been aggres-*

sive to people and animals, destroyed property, deceived other peo-
ple, or stolen things?

   If yes, ask: *Have these behaviors ever caused you significant*
trouble with your friends or family, at school or work, with the au-
thorities, or in another setting?

- If persistent anger or argumentativeness predominates, proceed to oppositional defiant disorder criteria.
- If recurrent behavioral outbursts predominate, proceed to intermittent explosive disorder criteria.
- If recurrent rule breaking predominates, proceed to conduct disorder criteria.

1. Oppositional Defiant Disorder [313.81, 462–466]

This section contains questions phrased for interviewing an older child with an ability to self-reflect. For younger children or those with limited cognitive functioning, rephrase these questions to interview the child's caregiver instead.

   a. Inclusion: Requires a pattern of at least <u>four</u> of the following angry, argumentative, or vindictive behaviors with nonsiblings over the course of more than 6 months:

   Angry/irritable mood

   i.   Often loses temper: *Do you often get explosively mad at people? Does your getting really mad cause you more problems?*
   ii. Often touchy or easily annoyed: *Do you get annoyed really easily by other people?*
   iii. Often angry and resentful: *Do you feel angry much of the time? Do you often feel people are making your life difficult?*

   Argumentative/defiant behavior

   i.   Often argues with adults: *Do you often get in arguments with your parents or teachers?*
   ii. Often actively defies rules or requests from authorities: *Do you often push back against rules or expectations?*
   iii. Often deliberately annoys others: *Do you often push other people's buttons just to get them to react?*
   iv. Often blames others for own mistakes or misbehaviors: *When you get caught doing something you*

aren't supposed to, are you likely to say it was someone else's fault?

Vindictiveness

i. Has been spiteful or vindictive twice or more in past 6 months: *Have you planned to get back at people you think have wronged you and then acted on that plan?*

b. Inclusion: Behavior disturbance causes distress in individual or others in their immediate social context or impacts functioning.

c. Exclusion: Problem does not exclusively occur from psychosis, substance abuse, depression, bipolar disorder, or disruptive mood dysregulation disorder.

2. Intermittent Explosive Disorder [F63.81, 466–469]

a. Inclusion: Requires recurrent behavioral outbursts in which a young person does not control aggressive impulses as manifested by <u>either</u> of the following.

i. Verbal or physical aggression: *Over the past 3 months, have you had impulsive outbursts in which you were verbally or physically aggressive toward other people, animals, or property? Have these outbursts occurred, on average, at least twice weekly?*

ii. Three behavioral outbursts involving damage to or destruction of property and/or physical assault: *Over the last 12 months, have you assaulted other people or destroyed property three or more times? Over the last 3 months, have you also had at least one impulsive outburst when you lost control of your behavior?*

b. Inclusion: Also requires all <u>three</u> of the following.

i. Magnitude of aggressiveness is disproportionate to any provocation or psychosocial stressor: *If you look back at these outbursts, can you identify any events or stressors that you associate with them? Was your response much more aggressive or extreme than these events or stressors?*

ii. Recurrent outbursts are neither premeditated nor in pursuit of a tangible objective: *When you had these outbursts, did they happen when you were feeling angry or impulsive? Did the outburst occur without a clear goal such as obtaining money or intimidating someone?*

iii. Outbursts cause marked personal distress, impair function, or are associated with financial or legal consequences: *How do these outbursts affect how you feel about yourself and how you get along with friends, family, and other people in your life? Have you ever suffered financial or legal consequences because of your outbursts?*

c. Exclusions

i. If a young person's chronological age, or equivalent developmental age, is younger than 6 years, do not use this diagnosis.

ii. If the recurrent aggressive outbursts are fully explained by another mental disorder or are attributable to another medical condition or to the physiological effects of a substance/medication, do not use this diagnosis.

iii. If aggressive behavior occurs only in the context of an adjustment disorder, do not use this diagnosis.

3. Conduct Disorder [F91.x, 469–475]

a. Inclusion: Requires a repetitive and persistent pattern of behavior in which the basic rights of others or major age-appropriate societal norms or rules are violated, as manifested by the presence of at least <u>three</u> of the following in the past 12 months and at least <u>one</u> of the following in the past 6 months.

i. Often bullies, threatens, or intimidates others: *Do you often bully, threaten, or intimidate other people?*

ii. Often initiates physical fights: *Do you often start physical fights?*

iii. Has used a weapon that can cause serious physical harm to others: *Have you used a weapon that could cause serious harm to someone else, such as a bat, brick, broken bottle, knife, or gun?*

iv. Has been physically cruel to people: *Have you caused physical pain or suffering to other people?*

v. Has been physically cruel to animals: *Have you caused physical pain or suffering to animals?*

vi. Has stolen while confronting a victim: *Have you forcibly taken or stolen something from someone while the person was present?*

vii. Has forced someone into sexual activity: *Have you forced someone into sexual activity?*

viii. Has deliberately engaged in fire setting with the intention of causing serious damage: *Have you set fires in order to cause serious damage to a person, animal, or property?*

ix. Has deliberated destroyed others' property: *Have you deliberately destroyed someone else's belongings?*

x. Has broken into someone else's house, building, or car: *Have you broken into someone else's house, building, or car?*

xi. Often lies to obtain goods or favors or to avoid obligations: *Do you often lie to get out of school or work or to get things you want?*

xii. Has stolen items of nontrivial value without confronting a victim: *Have you taken or stolen something valuable from someone when the person was not present?*

xiii. Often stays out at night despite parental prohibitions, beginning before age 13: *Before age 13, did you have a curfew, a time after which you had to be at home, that you often violated by staying out later than you were supposed to?*

xiv. Has run away from home overnight at least twice while living in parental or parental surrogate home (or once without returning for a lengthy period): *Have you ever run away from home? How many times? Did you ever run away from home without returning for a long time?*

xv. Is often truant from school, beginning before age 13: *Before age 13, did you often cut class or skip school?*

b. Modifiers

i. Specifiers

- Childhood-onset type [F91.1, 470]: Use when at least one criterion symptom begins before age 10 years.

- Adolescent-onset type [F91.2, 470]: Use when no criteria symptoms are present before age 10 years.

- Unspecified onset [F91.9, 470]: Use when the age at onset is unknown.

- With limited prosocial emotions: Use for a young person who persistently has at least <u>two</u> of the following characteristics: lack of remorse or guilt, callous lack of empathy, lack of concern about performance, and shallow or deficient affect. To meet criteria, these characteristics must be seen in multiple relationships and settings over at least 12 months. That is, these characteristics reflect a person's typical pattern of interpersonal and emotional functioning and not just occasional occurrences in some situations.

  ii. Severity

  • Mild: Few, if any, conduct problems beyond those required for diagnosis and relatively minor harm to others
  • Moderate
  • Severe: Many conduct problems beyond those required for diagnosis, or considerable harm to others

c. Alternatives

  i. If a young person shows at least 6 months of a persistent pattern of angry and irritable mood along with defiant and vindictive behavior, consider oppositional defiant disorder [F91.3, 462–466]. The pattern is manifested by at least <u>four</u> of the following: often losing temper, being touchy or easily annoyed by others, being angry and resentful, arguing with adults, actively defying or refusing to comply with adults' requests or rules, deliberately annoying people, blaming others for one's mistakes or misbehaviors, or being spiteful or vindictive at least twice within the past 6 months. In addition, it is important to consider the persistence and frequency of these behaviors in relation to a person's developmental stage. For children younger than age 5, the behavior must occur on most days for at least 6 months. For children age 5 years or older, the behavior must occur at least once a week for at least 6 months. The behaviors must also cause clinically significant impairment and cannot occur exclusively during the course of a psychotic, substance use, depressive, or bipolar disorder, and the criteria for disruptive mood dysregulation disorder cannot be met.

  ii. If a young person reports deliberate and purposeful fire setting on at least two occasions, consider pyromania [F63.1, 476–477]. The diagnosis requires tension or affective arousal before the fire setting, fascination with fire, and pleasure or relief when setting or witnessing fires. If the fire setting is done for monetary gain, to conceal criminal activity, out of anger, or in response to a hallucination, do not use this diagnosis. If the fire setting is better explained by intellectual disability, conduct disorder, mania, or antisocial personality disorder, do not use this diagnosis.

iii. If a young person repeatedly fails to resist impulses to steal objects that are not needed for his personal use or their monetary value, consider kleptomania [F63.2, 478–479]. The diagnosis requires tension or affective arousal before the theft and pleasure or relief at the time of the theft. If the stealing is done out of anger or vengeance or in response to a hallucination, do not use this diagnosis. If the stealing is better explained by conduct disorder, mania, or antisocial personality disorder, do not use this diagnosis.

iv. If a young person has symptoms characteristic of a disruptive, impulse-control, and conduct disorder that cause clinically significant distress or impairment without meeting the full criteria for a diagnosis named earlier, consider unspecified disruptive, impulse-control, and conduct disorder [F91.9, 480]. If you wish to communicate the specific reason that a young person does not meet the full criteria, consider other specified disruptive, impulse-control, and conduct disorder [F91.8, 479].

Substance-Related and Addictive Disorders

DSM-5 pp. 481–589

Screening question: *In the past year, have you drunk alcohol, smoked marijuana, or used anything else to get high? Have you ever ridden in a car with someone who was high or drinking alcohol? Do you ever use alcohol or drugs when you are alone? Do you ever use alcohol or drugs to relax?* (Knight et al. 2002)

If yes, ask: *Did these experiences ever cause you significant trouble with your friends or family, at school, or in another setting?*

- If a young person reports problems with substance use, proceed to the substance use disorder criteria for each particular substance.
- If a young person presents with substance intoxication, proceed to the substance intoxication criteria for each particular substance.
- If a young person reports problems with substance withdrawal, proceed to the substance withdrawal criteria for each particular substance.

1. Alcohol Use Disorder [F10.x0, 490–497]

   a. Inclusion: Requires a problematic pattern of alcohol use leading to clinically significant impairment or distress as manifested by at least <u>two</u> of the following symptoms in a 12-month period.

      i. Drinking more alcohol over a longer period than intended: *When you drink, do you find that you drink more, and for a longer time, than you planned to?*

      ii. Persistent desire or unsuccessful effort to reduce alcohol use: *Do you want to cut back or stop drinking? Have you ever tried and failed to cut back or stop drinking?*

      iii. Great deal of time spent: *Do you spend a great deal of your time obtaining alcohol, drinking alcohol, or recovering from your alcohol use?*

      iv. Cravings: *Do you experience strong desires or cravings to drink alcohol?*

      v. Failure to fulfill major role obligations: *Have you repeatedly failed to fulfill major obligations at home, school, or work because of your alcohol use?*

      vi. Continued use despite awareness of interpersonal or social problems: *Do you drink alcohol even though you suspect, or even know, that it creates or worsens interpersonal or social problems?*

      vii. Giving up activities for alcohol: *Are there important social, occupational, or recreational activities that you have given up or reduced because of your alcohol use?*

      viii. Use in hazardous situations: *Have you repeatedly used alcohol in situations in which it was physically hazardous, such as driving a car or operating a machine while intoxicated?*

      ix. Continued use despite awareness of physical or psychological problems: *Do you drink alcohol even though you suspect, or even know, that it creates or worsens problems with your mind and body?*

 x. Tolerance as manifested by <u>either</u> of the following.

- Markedly increased amounts: *Do you find that in order to get intoxicated or achieve the desired effect of drinking, you need to consume much more alcohol than you used to?*
- Markedly diminished effects: *If you drink the same amount of alcohol as you used to, do you find that it has a lot less effect on you than it used to?*

 xi. Withdrawal as manifested by <u>either</u> of the following.

- Characteristic alcohol withdrawal syndrome: *When you stop drinking, do you undergo withdrawal?*
- The same or closely related substance is taken to relieve or avoid withdrawal symptoms: *Have you ever drunk alcohol or taken another substance to prevent alcohol withdrawal?*

b. Modifiers

 i. Specifiers

- In early remission
- In sustained remission
- In a controlled environment

 ii. Severity

- Mild [F10.10, 491]: use when two to three symptoms are present
- Moderate [F10.20, 491]: use when four to five symptoms are present
- Severe [F10.20, 491]: use when six or more symptoms are present

c. Alternatives

 i. If a young person received more than minimal exposure to alcohol at any time during gestation and subsequently experiences neurocognitive impairment, impaired self-regulation, and deficits in adaptive functioning, consider neurobehavioral disorder associated with prenatal alcohol exposure and other specified neurodevelopmental disorder [F88, 86]. The prenatal exposure results in symptoms beginning before age 18 years that result in clinically significant distress or functional impairment.

ii. If a young person experiences problems associated with the use of alcohol that are not classifiable as alcohol use disorder, alcohol intoxication, alcohol withdrawal, alcohol intoxication delirium, alcohol withdrawal delirium, alcohol-induced neurocognitive disorder, alcohol-induced psychotic disorder, alcohol-induced bipolar disorder, alcohol-induced depressive disorder, alcohol-induced anxiety disorder, alcohol-induced sexual dysfunction, or alcohol-induced sleep disorder, consider unspecified alcohol-related disorder [F10.99, 503].

2. Alcohol Intoxication [F10.x29, 497–499]

a. Inclusion: Requires at least <u>one</u> of the following signs or symptoms developing during, or shortly after, alcohol use.

i. Slurred speech
ii. Incoordination
iii. Unsteady gait
iv. Nystagmus
v. Impairment in attention or memory
vi. Stupor or coma

b. Inclusion: Requires clinically significant problematic behavioral or psychological changes. *Since you began this episode of drinking, have you observed any significant changes in your behavior, mood, or judgment? Have you engaged in problematic activities or thought problematic thoughts that you would not have if you were sober?*

c. Exclusion: If the symptoms are attributable to another medical condition or are better explained by another mental disorder, including intoxication with another substance, do not use this diagnosis.

3. Alcohol Withdrawal [F10.23x, 499–501]

a. Inclusion: Requires at least <u>two</u> of the following symptoms developing within several hours to a few days of ceasing (or reducing) alcohol use that has been heavy and prolonged.

i. Autonomic hyperactivity
ii. Increased hand tremor

iii. Insomnia: *Over the last couple of days, have you found it more difficult than usual to get to sleep and to stay asleep?*

iv. Nausea or vomiting: *Over the last couple of days, have you felt sick to your stomach, felt nauseated, or even vomited?*

v. Transient visual, tactile, or auditory hallucinations or illusions: *Over the last couple of days, have you had any experiences where you worried that your mind was playing tricks on you, such as seeing, hearing, or feeling things that other people could not?*

vi. Psychomotor agitation

vii. Anxiety: *Over the last couple of days, have you felt more worried or anxious than usual?*

viii. Generalized tonic-clonic seizures

b. Exclusion: If the symptoms are attributable to another medical condition or are better explained by another mental disorder, including intoxication with or withdrawal from another substance, do not use this diagnosis.

c. Modifiers

i. Specifier

- With perceptual disturbances [F10.232, 500]

4. Caffeine Intoxication [F15.929, 503–506]

a. Inclusion: Requires clinically significant problematic behavioral or psychological changes shortly after caffeine ingestion, usually in excess of 250 mg (e.g., 2–3 cups of brewed coffee), as manifested by at least <u>five</u> of the following signs or symptoms.

i. Restlessness: *Over the last several hours, have you felt less able to remain at rest than usual?*

ii. Nervousness: *Over the last several hours, have you felt more jittery or nervous than usual?*

iii. Excitement: *Over the last several hours, have you felt more excited than usual?*

iv. Insomnia: *Over the last several hours, if you tried to sleep, did you find it more difficult to get to sleep or stay asleep than usual?*

v. Flushed face

vi. Diuresis: *Over the last several hours, have you urinated more often or a greater amount than usual?*

vii. Gastrointestinal disturbance: *Over the last several hours, have you experienced an upset stomach, nausea, vomiting, or diarrhea?*

viii. Muscle twitching: *Over the last several hours, have you noticed your muscles twitching more than usual?*

ix. Rambling flow of thought and speech: *Over the last several hours, have you or anyone else noticed that your thoughts or speech have been long winded or even confused?*

x. Tachycardia or cardiac arrhythmia

xi. Periods of inexhaustibility: *Over the last several hours, have you felt as if you had so much energy it could not be used up?*

xii. Psychomotor agitation

b. Exclusion: If the symptoms are attributable to another medical condition or are better explained by another mental disorder, including intoxication with another substance, do not use this diagnosis.

c. Alternative: If a person experiences problems associated with the use of caffeine that are not classifiable as caffeine intoxication, caffeine withdrawal, caffeine-induced anxiety disorder, or caffeine-induced sleep disorder, consider unspecified caffeine-related disorder [F15.99, 509].

5. Caffeine Withdrawal [F15.93, 506–508]

a. Inclusion: Requires at least <u>three</u> of the following symptoms developing within 24 hours of ceasing (or reducing) caffeine use that has been prolonged.

i. Headache: *Over the last day, have you had any headaches?*

ii. Marked fatigue or drowsiness: *Over the last day, have you felt extremely tired or sleepy?*

iii. Dysphoric or depressed mood or irritability: *Over the last day, have you felt more down, more depressed, or even more irritable than usual?*

iv. Difficulty concentrating: *Over the last day, have you had difficulty staying focused on a task or an activity?*

v. Flulike symptoms: *Over the last day, have you experienced flulike symptoms, nausea, vomiting, or muscle pain or stiffness?*

b. Exclusion: If the symptoms are attributable to another medical condition or are better explained by another mental disorder, including intoxication with or withdrawal from another substance, do not use this diagnosis.

6. Cannabis Use Disorder [F12.x0, 509–516]

a. Inclusion: Requires a problematic pattern of cannabis use leading to clinically significant impairment or distress as manifested by at least two of the following in a 12-month period.

   i. Consuming more cannabis over a longer period than intended: *When you use cannabis, do you find that you use more, and for a longer time, than you planned to?*

   ii. Persistent desire or unsuccessful effort to reduce cannabis use: *Do you want to cut back or stop using cannabis? Have you ever tried and failed to cut back or stop?*

   iii. Great deal of time spent: *Do you spend a great deal of your time obtaining cannabis, using cannabis, or recovering from your cannabis use?*

   iv. Cravings: *Do you experience strong desires or cravings to use cannabis?*

   v. Failure to fulfill major role obligations: *Have you repeatedly failed to fulfill major obligations at home, school, or work because of your cannabis use?*

   vi. Continued use despite awareness of interpersonal or social problems: *Do you use cannabis even though you suspect, or even know, that it creates or worsens interpersonal or social problems?*

   vii. Giving up activities for cannabis: *Are there important social, occupational, or recreational activities that you have given up or reduced because of your cannabis use?*

   viii. Use in hazardous situations: *Have you repeatedly used cannabis in situations in which it was physically hazardous, such as driving a car or operating a machine while intoxicated?*

   ix. Continued use despite awareness of physical or psychological problems: *Do you use cannabis even though you suspect, or even know, that it creates or worsens problems with your mind and body?*

   x. Tolerance as manifested by either of the following.

   • Markedly increased amounts: *Do you find that in order to get high or achieve the desired effect of using cannabis, you need to smoke or ingest much more cannabis than you used to?*

- Markedly diminished effects: *If you use the same amount of cannabis as you used to, do you find that it has a lot less effect on you than it used to?*

xi. Withdrawal as manifested by <u>either</u> of the following.

- Characteristic cannabis withdrawal syndrome: *When you stop using cannabis, do you undergo withdrawal?*
- The same or related substance is taken to relieve or avoid withdrawal symptoms: *Have you used cannabis or another substance to prevent yourself from withdrawing from cannabis?*

b. Modifiers

i. Specifiers

- In early remission
- In sustained remission
- In a controlled environment

ii. Severity

- Mild [F12.10, 510]: use when two or three symptoms are present
- Moderate [F12.20, 510]: use when four or five symptoms are present
- Severe [F12.20, 510]: use when six or more symptoms are present

c. Alternative: If a young person experiences problems associated with the use of cannabis that are not classifiable as cannabis use disorder, cannabis intoxication, cannabis withdrawal, cannabis intoxication delirium, cannabis withdrawal delirium, cannabis-induced neurocognitive disorder, cannabis-induced psychotic disorder, cannabis-induced bipolar disorder, cannabis-induced depressive disorder, cannabis-induced anxiety disorder, cannabis-induced sexual dysfunction, or cannabis-induced sleep disorder, consider unspecified cannabis-related disorder [F12.99, 519].

7. Cannabis Intoxication [F12.x2x, 516–517]

a. Inclusion: Requires at least <u>two</u> of the following signs or symptoms shortly after cannabis use.

i. Conjunctival injection

ii. Increased appetite: *Over the last several hours, have you been much hungrier than usual?*

iii. Dry mouth: *Over the last several hours, have you noticed that your mouth has been dry?*

iv. Tachycardia

b. Inclusion: Requires clinically significant problematic behavioral or psychological changes. *Since you began this episode of cannabis use, have you observed any significant changes in your mood, judgment, ability to interact with others, or sense of time? Have you engaged in problematic activities, or thought problematic thoughts, that you would not have without cannabis?*

c. Exclusion: If the symptoms are attributable to another medical condition or are better explained by another mental disorder, including intoxication with another substance, do not use this diagnosis.

d. Modifiers

i. Specifier

- With perceptual disturbance [F12.x22, 516]

8. Cannabis Withdrawal [F12.288, 517–519]

a. Inclusion: Requires at least <u>three</u> of the following symptoms developing within 1 week of ceasing (or reducing) cannabis use that has been heavy and prolonged.

i. Irritability, anger, or aggression: *Over the last week or so, have you felt more irritable or angry or that you were ready to confront or attack someone?*

ii. Nervousness or anxiety: *Over the last week or so, have you felt more worried or anxious than usual?*

iii. Sleep difficulty: *Over the last week or so, have you had any disturbing dreams or found it more difficult to get to sleep and to stay asleep than usual?*

iv. Decreased appetite or weight loss: *Over the last week or so, have you been less hungry or even lost weight?*

v. Restlessness: *Over the last week or so, have you felt less able to remain at rest than usual?*

vi. Depressed mood: *Over the last week or so, have you felt more down or depressed than usual?*

vii. Somatic symptoms: *Over the last week or so, have you felt any unusual physical discomfort, such as stomach pain, tremors, sweating, fever, chills, or headaches?*

b. Exclusion: If the symptoms are attributable to another medical condition or are better explained by another mental disorder, including intoxication with or withdrawal from another substance, do not use this diagnosis.

9. Phencyclidine or Other Hallucinogen Use Disorder [F16.x0, 520–527]

   a. Inclusion: Requires a problematic pattern of phencyclidine or other hallucinogen use leading to clinically significant impairment or distress as manifested by at least <u>two</u> of the following in a 12-month period.

   i. Using more phencyclidine or other hallucinogens over a longer period than intended: *When you use hallucinogens, do you find that you use more, and for a longer time, than you planned to?*

   ii. Persistent desire or unsuccessful effort to reduce hallucinogen use: *Do you want to cut back or stop using hallucinogens? Have you ever tried and failed to cut back or stop using hallucinogens?*

   iii. Great deal of time spent: *Do you spend a great deal of your time obtaining hallucinogens, using hallucinogens, or recovering from your hallucinogen use?*

   iv. Cravings: *Do you experience strong desires or cravings to use hallucinogens?*

   v. Failure to fulfill major role obligations: *Have you repeatedly failed to fulfill major obligations at home, school, or work because of your hallucinogen use?*

   vi. Continued use despite awareness of interpersonal or social problems: *Do you use hallucinogens even though you suspect, or even know, that your use creates or worsens interpersonal or social problems?*

   vii. Giving up activities for hallucinogens: *Are there important social, occupational, or recreational activities that you have given up or reduced because of your hallucinogen use?*

   viii. Use in hazardous situations: *Have you repeatedly used hallucinogens in situations in which it was physically hazardous, such as driving a car or operating a machine while intoxicated?*

   ix. Continued use despite awareness of physical or psychological problems: *Do you use hallucinogens even though you suspect, or even know, that they create or worsen problems with your mind and body?*

   x. Tolerance as manifested by <u>either</u> of the following.

- Markedly increased amounts: *Do you find that in order to achieve the desired effect of hallucinogens, you need to consume much more than you used to?*
- Markedly diminished effects: *If you use the same amount of a hallucinogen as you used to, do you find that it has a lot less effect on you than it used to?*

b. Modifiers

i. Specifiers
- In early remission
- In sustained remission
- In a controlled environment

ii. Severity
- Mild [F16.10, 521/524]: use when two or three symptoms are present
- Moderate [F16.20, 521/524]: use when four or five symptoms are present
- Severe [F16.20, 521/524]: use when six or more symptoms are present

c. Alternative: If a young person experiences problems associated with the use of phencyclidine or other hallucinogens that are not classifiable as phencyclidine or other hallucinogen use disorder, phencyclidine or other hallucinogen intoxication, phencyclidine or other hallucinogen withdrawal, phencyclidine or other hallucinogen intoxication delirium, phencyclidine or other hallucinogen withdrawal delirium, phencyclidine- or other hallucinogen-induced neurocognitive disorder, phencyclidine- or other hallucinogen-induced psychotic disorder, phencyclidine- or other hallucinogen-induced bipolar disorder, phencyclidine- or other hallucinogen-induced depressive disorder, phencyclidine- or other hallucinogen-induced anxiety disorder, phencyclidine- or other hallucinogen-induced sexual dysfunction, or phencyclidine- or other hallucinogen-induced sleep disorder, consider unspecified phencyclidine-related disorder or unspecified hallucinogen-related disorder [F16.99, 533].

10. Phencyclidine or Other Hallucinogen Intoxication [F16.x29, 527–530]

a. Inclusion: Requires at least two of the following signs during or shortly after hallucinogen use.

Phencyclidine

    i. Vertical or horizontal nystagmus

   ii. Hypertension or tachycardia

  iii. Numbness or diminished responsiveness to pain

   iv. Ataxia

    v. Dysarthria

   vi. Muscle rigidity

  vii. Seizures or coma

 viii. Hyperacusis

Other Hallucinogens

    i. Pupillary dilation

   ii. Tachycardia

  iii. Sweating: *Since taking the hallucinogen, have you noticed any change in how much you sweat?*

   iv. Palpitations: *Since taking the hallucinogen, has your heartbeat been more rapid, strong, or irregular than usual?*

    v. Blurring of vision: *Since taking the hallucinogen, has your vision been blurred?*

   vi. Tremors

  vii. Incoordination: *Since taking the hallucinogen, have you found it hard to coordinate your movements as you walk or otherwise move?*

b. Inclusion: Requires clinically significant problematic behavioral or psychological changes. *Since you began this episode of hallucinogen use, have you observed any significant changes in your mood, judgment, ability to interact with others, or sense of time? Have you engaged in problematic activities, or thought problematic thoughts, that you would not have without hallucinogens?*

c. Exclusion: If the symptoms are attributable to another medical condition or are better explained by another mental disorder, including intoxication with another substance, do not use this diagnosis.

11. Inhalant Use Disorder [F18.x0, 533–538]

a. Inclusion: Requires a problematic pattern of inhalant use leading to clinically significant impairment or distress as manifested by at least <u>two</u> of the following in a 12-month period.

    i. Using more inhalants over a longer period than intended: *When you inhale, do you find that you use more inhalant, and for a longer time, than you planned to?*

ii. Persistent desire or unsuccessful effort to reduce inhalant use: *Do you want to cut back or stop inhaling? Have you ever tried and failed to cut back or stop inhaling?*

iii. Great deal of time spent: *Do you spend a great deal of your time obtaining inhalants, using inhalants, or recovering from your inhalant use?*

iv. Cravings: *Do you experience strong desires or cravings to use inhalants?*

v. Failure to fulfill major role obligations: *Have you repeatedly failed to fulfill major obligations at home, school, or work because of your inhalant use?*

vi. Continued use despite awareness of interpersonal or social problems: *Do you use inhalants even though you suspect, or even know, that your use creates or worsens interpersonal or social problems?*

vii. Giving up activities for inhalants: *Are there important social, occupational, or recreational activities that you have given up or reduced because of your inhalant use?*

viii. Use in hazardous situations: *Have you repeatedly used inhalants in situations in which it was physically hazardous, such as driving a car or operating a machine while high?*

ix. Continued use despite awareness of physical or psychological problems: *Do you use inhalants even though you suspect, or even know, that it creates or worsens problems with your mind and body?*

x. Tolerance as manifested by <u>either</u> of the following.

- Markedly increased amounts: *Do you find that in order to get high or achieve the desired effect of using inhalants, you need to use much more than you used to?*
- Markedly diminished effects: *If you inhale the same amount of an inhalant as you used to, do you find that it has a lot less effect on you than it used to?*

b. Modifiers

i. Specifiers
- In early remission
- In sustained remission
- In a controlled environment

ii. Severity
- Mild [F18.10, 534]: use when two or three symptoms are present

- Moderate [F18.20, 534]: use when four or five symptoms are present
- Severe [F18.20, 534]: use when six or more symptoms are present

c. Alternative: If a young person experiences problems associated with the use of an inhalant that are not classifiable as inhalant use disorder, inhalant intoxication, inhalant withdrawal, inhalant intoxication delirium, inhalant withdrawal delirium, inhalant-induced neurocognitive disorder, inhalant-induced psychotic disorder, inhalant-induced bipolar disorder, inhalant-induced depressive disorder, inhalant-induced anxiety disorder, inhalant-induced sexual dysfunction, or inhalant-induced sleep disorder, consider unspecified inhalant-related disorder [F18.99, 540].

12. Inhalant Intoxication [F18.x29, 538–540]

a. Inclusion: Requires at least <u>two</u> of the following signs or symptoms after intended or unintended short-term, high-dose inhalant exposure.

  i. Dizziness: *Since using the inhalant, have you felt like you were reeling or about to fall?*
  ii. Nystagmus
  iii. Incoordination: *Since using the inhalant, have you found it hard to coordinate your movements as you walk or otherwise move?*
  iv. Slurred speech
  v. Unsteady gait
  vi. Lethargy: *Since using the inhalant, have you felt very sleepy or a marked lack of energy?*
  vii. Depressed reflexes
  viii. Psychomotor retardation
  ix. Tremor
  x. Generalized muscle weakness
  xi. Blurred vision or diplopia: *Since using the inhalant, has your vision been blurred, or have you been seeing double?*
  xii. Stupor or coma
  xiii. Euphoria: *Since using the inhalant, have you felt mentally or physically elated or intensely excited or happy?*

b. Inclusion: Requires clinically significant problematic behavioral or psychological changes. *Since you began this episode of inhalant use, have you observed any signifi-*

cant changes in your mood, judgment, ability to interact with others, or sense of time? Have you engaged in problematic activities, or thought problematic thoughts, that you would not have without inhalants?

    c. Exclusion: If the symptoms are attributable to another medical condition or are better explained by another mental disorder, including intoxication with another substance, do not use this diagnosis.

13. Opioid Use Disorder [F11.x0, 541–546]

    a. Inclusion: Requires a maladaptive pattern of opioid use leading to clinically significant impairment or distress as manifested by at least <u>two</u> of the following in a 12-month period.

        i. Using more opioids over a longer period than intended: *When you use opioids, do you find that you use more, and for a longer time, than you planned to?*

        ii. Persistent desire or unsuccessful effort to reduce opioid use: *Do you want to cut back or stop using opioids? Have you ever tried and failed to cut back or stop your opioid use?*

        iii. Great deal of time spent: *Do you spend a great deal of your time obtaining opioids, using opioids, or recovering from your opioid use?*

        iv. Cravings: *Do you experience strong desires or cravings to use opioids?*

        v. Failure to fulfill major role obligations: *Have you repeatedly failed to fulfill major obligations at home, school, or work because of your opioid use?*

        vi. Continued use despite awareness of interpersonal or social problems: *Do you continue to use opioids even though you suspect, or even know, that your use creates or worsens interpersonal or social problems?*

        vii. Giving up activities for opioids: *Are there important social, occupational, or recreational activities that you have given up or reduced because of your opioid use?*

        viii. Use in hazardous situations: *Have you repeatedly used opioids in situations in which it was physically hazardous, such as driving a car or operating a machine while intoxicated?*

        ix. Continued use despite awareness of physical or psychological problems: *Do you use opioids even though you suspect, or even know, that it creates or worsens problems with your mind and body?*

x. Tolerance as manifested by <u>either</u> of the following.

- Markedly increased amounts: *Do you find that in order to get high or achieve the desired effect of using opioids, you need to consume much more than you used to?*
- Markedly diminished effects (excluding opioid medications taken under medical supervision): *If you use the same amount of an opioid as you used to, do you find that it has a lot less effect on you than it used to?*

xi. Withdrawal as manifested by <u>either</u> of the following.

- Characteristic opioid withdrawal syndrome: *When you stop using opioids, do you undergo withdrawal?*
- The same or closely related substance is taken to relieve or avoid withdrawal symptoms: *Have you ever taken opioids or another substance to prevent opioid withdrawal?*

b. Modifiers

   i. Specifiers

   - In early remission
   - In sustained remission
   - On maintenance therapy
   - In a controlled environment

   ii. Severity

   - Mild [F11.10, 542]: use when two or three symptoms are present
   - Moderate [F11.20, 542]: use when four or five symptoms are present
   - Severe [F11.20, 542]: use when six or more symptoms are present

c. Alternative: If a young person experiences problems associated with the use of opioids that are not classifiable as opioid use disorder, opioid intoxication, opioid withdrawal, opioid intoxication delirium, opioid withdrawal delirium, opioid-induced neurocognitive disorder, opioid-induced psychotic disorder, opioid-induced bipolar disorder, opioid-induced depressive disorder, opioid-induced anxiety disorder, opioid-induced sexual dysfunction, or opioid-induced sleep disorder, consider unspecified opioid-related disorder [F11.99, 550].

14. Opioid Intoxication [F11.x2x, 546–547]

  a. Inclusion: Requires pupillary constriction shortly after opioid use and at least <u>one</u> of the following signs.

    i. Drowsiness or coma
    ii. Slurred speech
    iii. Impairment in attention or memory

  b. Inclusion: Requires clinically significant problematic behavioral or psychological changes. *Since you began this episode of opioid use, have you observed any significant changes in your mood, judgment, ability to interact with others, or sense of time? Have you engaged in problematic activities, or thought problematic thoughts, that you would not have without opioids?*

  c. Exclusion: If the symptoms are attributable to another medical condition or are better explained by another mental disorder, including intoxication with another substance, do not use this diagnosis.

  d. Modifiers

    i. Specifier

      • With perceptual disturbance [F11.x22, 546–547]

15. Opioid Withdrawal [F11.23, 547–549]

  a. Inclusion: Requires at least <u>three</u> of the following symptoms developing within minutes to several days of ceasing (or reducing) opioid use that has been heavy and prolonged OR following the administration of an opioid antagonist after a period of opioid use.

    i. Dysphoric mood: *Over the last couple of days, have you been feeling more down or depressed than usual?*
    ii. Nausea or vomiting: *Over the last couple of days, have you felt sick to your stomach, felt nauseated, or even vomited?*
    iii. Muscle aches: *Over the last couple of days, have you experienced muscle aches or pains?*
    iv. Lacrimation or rhinorrhea: *Over the last couple of days, have you noticed that you have been shedding tears when you did not feel like crying? Have you no-*

ticed that your nose has been running, or discharging clear fluid, more than usual?

   v. Pupillary dilation, piloerection, or sweating

  vi. Diarrhea: *Over the last couple of days, have you experienced more frequent or more liquid stools than usual?*

 vii. Yawning: *Over the last couple of days, have you been yawning much more than usual?*

viii. Fever

  ix. Insomnia: *Over the last couple of days, have you found it more difficult than usual to get to sleep and to stay asleep?*

b. Exclusion: If the symptoms are attributable to another medical condition or are better explained by another mental disorder, including intoxication with or withdrawal from another substance, do not use this diagnosis.

16. Sedative, Hypnotic, or Anxiolytic Use Disorder [F13.x0, 550–556]

a. Inclusion: Requires a problematic pattern of sedative, hypnotic, or anxiolytic use leading to clinically significant impairment or distress as manifested by at least <u>two</u> of the following in a 12-month period.

    i. Using more sedatives, hypnotics, or anxiolytics over a longer period than intended: *When you use sedatives, hypnotics, or anxiolytics, do you find that you use more, and for a longer time, than you planned to?*

   ii. Persistent desire or unsuccessful effort to reduce sedative, hypnotic, or anxiolytic use: *Do you want to cut back or stop using sedatives, hypnotics, or anxiolytics? Have you ever tried and failed to cut back or stop using sedatives, hypnotics, or anxiolytics?*

  iii. Great deal of time spent: *Do you spend a great deal of your time obtaining and using sedatives, hypnotics,* or anxiolytics *or recovering from your sedative, hypnotic, or anxiolytic use?*

  iv. Cravings: *Do you experience strong desires or cravings to use sedatives, hypnotics, or anxiolytics?*

   v. Failure to fulfill major role obligations: *Have you repeatedly failed to fulfill major obligations at home, school, or work because of your sedative, hypnotic, or anxiolytic use?*

  vi. Continued use despite awareness of interpersonal or social problems: *Do you use a sedative, hypnotic, or anxiolytic even though you suspect, or even know, that it creates or worsens interpersonal or social problems?*

vii. Giving up activities for sedatives, hypnotics, or anxiolytics: *Are there important social, occupational, or recreational activities that you have given up or reduced because of your sedative, hypnotic, or anxiolytic use?*

viii. Use in hazardous situations: *Have you repeatedly used a sedative, hypnotic, or anxiolytic in situations in which it was physically hazardous, such as driving a car or operating a machine while intoxicated?*

ix. Continued use despite awareness of physical or psychological problems: *Do you use sedatives, hypnotics, or anxiolytics even though you suspect, or even know, that your use creates or worsens problems with your mind and body?*

x. Tolerance as manifested by <u>either</u> of the following.

- Markedly increased amounts: *Do you find that in order to get intoxicated or achieve the desired effect of using sedatives, hypnotics, or anxiolytics, you need to consume much more than you used to?*
- Markedly diminished effects: *If you use the same amount of a sedative, hypnotic, or anxiolytic as you used to, do you find that it has a lot less effect on you than it used to?*

xi. Withdrawal as manifested by <u>either</u> of the following.

- Characteristic sedative, hypnotic, or anxiolytic withdrawal syndrome: *When you stop using sedatives, hypnotics, or anxiolytics, do you undergo withdrawal?*
- The same or closely related substance is taken to relieve or avoid withdrawal symptoms: *Have you ever taken sedatives, hypnotics, anxiolytics, or another substance to prevent withdrawal?*

b. Modifiers

i. Specifiers

- In early remission
- In sustained remission
- In a controlled environment

ii. Severity

- Mild [F13.10, 552]: use when two or three symptoms are present

- Moderate [F13.20, 552]: use when four or five symptoms are present
- Severe [F13.20, 552]: use when six or more symptoms are present

c. Alternative: If a young person experiences problems associated with the use of a sedative, hypnotic, or anxiolytic that are not classifiable as sedative, hypnotic, or anxiolytic use disorder; sedative, hypnotic, or anxiolytic intoxication; sedative, hypnotic, or anxiolytic withdrawal; sedative, hypnotic, or anxiolytic intoxication delirium; sedative, hypnotic, or anxiolytic withdrawal delirium; sedative-, hypnotic-, or anxiolytic-induced neurocognitive disorder; sedative-, hypnotic-, or anxiolytic-induced psychotic disorder; sedative-, hypnotic-, or anxiolytic-induced bipolar disorder; sedative-, hypnotic-, or anxiolytic-induced depressive disorder; sedative-, hypnotic-, or anxiolytic-induced anxiety disorder; sedative-, hypnotic-, or anxiolytic-induced sexual dysfunction; or sedative-, hypnotic-, or anxiolytic-induced sleep disorder, consider unspecified sedative-, hypnotic-, or anxiolytic-related disorder [F13.99, 560].

17. Sedative, Hypnotic, or Anxiolytic Intoxication [F13.x29, 556–557]

a. Inclusion: Requires <u>one</u> of the following signs shortly after sedative, hypnotic, or anxiolytic use.

i. Slurred speech
ii. Incoordination
iii. Unsteady gait
iv. Nystagmus
v. Impairment in cognition (i.e., attention or memory)
vi. Stupor or coma

b. Inclusion: Requires clinically significant problematic behavioral or psychological changes. *Since you began this episode of sedative, hypnotic, or anxiolytic use, have you observed any significant changes in your mood, judgment, ability to interact with others, or sense of time? Have you engaged in problematic activities, or thought problematic thoughts, that you would not have without the sedative, hypnotic, or anxiolytic?*

c. Exclusion: If the symptoms are attributable to another medical condition or are better explained by another mental disorder, including intoxication with another substance, do not use this diagnosis.

18. Sedative, Hypnotic, or Anxiolytic Withdrawal [F13.23x, 557–560]

    a. Inclusion: Requires at least <u>two</u> of the following symptoms developing within several hours to a few days after ceasing (or reducing) sedative, hypnotic, or anxiolytic use that has been heavy and prolonged.

        i. Autonomic hyperactivity

        ii. Hand tremor

        iii. Insomnia: *Over the last couple of days, have you found it more difficult than usual to get to sleep and to stay asleep?*

        iv. Nausea or vomiting: *Over the last couple of days, have you felt sick to your stomach, felt nauseated, or even vomited?*

        v. Transient visual, tactile, or auditory hallucinations or illusions: *Over the last couple of days, have you had any experiences where you worried that your mind was playing tricks on you, like seeing, hearing, or feeling things that other people could not?*

        vi. Psychomotor agitation

        vii. Anxiety: *Over the last couple of days, have you felt more worried or anxious than usual?*

        viii. Grand mal seizures

    b. Exclusion: If the symptoms are attributable to another medical condition or are better explained by another mental disorder, including intoxication with or withdrawal from another substance, do not use this diagnosis.

    c. Modifiers

        i. Specifier

          • With perceptual disturbances [F13.232, 558]

19. Stimulant Use Disorder [F1x.x0, 561–567]

    a. Inclusion: Requires a problematic pattern of stimulant use leading to clinically significant impairment or distress as manifested by at least <u>two</u> of the following in a 12-month period.

        i. Using more stimulants over a longer period than intended: *When you use stimulants, do you find that you use more, and for a longer time, than you planned to?*

ii. Persistent desire or unsuccessful effort to reduce stimulant use: *Do you want to cut back or stop using stimulants? Have you ever tried and failed to cut back or stop using stimulants?*

iii. Great deal of time spent: *Do you spend a great deal of your time obtaining stimulants, using stimulants, or recovering from your stimulant use?*

iv. Cravings: *Do you experience strong desires or cravings to use stimulants?*

v. Failure to fulfill major role obligations: *Have you repeatedly failed to fulfill major obligations at home, school, or work because of your stimulant use?*

vi. Continued use despite awareness of interpersonal or social problems: *Do you use stimulants even though you suspect, or even know, that your use creates or worsens interpersonal or social problems?*

vii. Giving up activities for stimulants: *Are there important social, occupational, or recreational activities that you have given up or reduced because of your stimulant use?*

viii. Use in hazardous situations: *Have you repeatedly used stimulants in situations in which it was physically hazardous, such as driving a car or operating a machine while intoxicated?*

ix. Continued use despite awareness of physical or psychological problems: *Do you use stimulants even though you suspect, or even know, that it creates or worsens problems with your mind and body?*

x. Tolerance as manifested by <u>either</u> of the following. **Note:** This criterion is not met if taking stimulants as prescribed under medical supervision.

- Markedly increased amounts: *Do you find that in order to get intoxicated or achieve the desired effect of using stimulants, you need to consume much more than you used to?*
- Markedly diminished effects (excluding stimulant medications taken under medical supervision to treat attention-deficit/hyperactivity disorder or narcolepsy): *If you use the same amount of a stimulant as you used to, do you find that it has a lot less effect on you than it used to?*

xi. Withdrawal as manifested by <u>either</u> of the following. **Note:** This criterion is not met if taking stimulants as prescribed under medical supervision.

- Characteristic stimulant withdrawal syndrome: *When you stop using stimulants, do you undergo withdrawal?*
- The same or a closely related substance is taken to relieve or avoid withdrawal symptoms (excluding stimulant medications taken under medical supervision to treat attention-deficit/hyperactivity disorder or narcolepsy): *Have you ever taken stimulants or another substance to prevent withdrawal?*

b. Modifiers

   i. Specify stimulant

   - Amphetamine-type substance
   - Cocaine
   - Other or unspecified stimulant

   ii. Specifiers

   - In early remission
   - In sustained remission
   - In a controlled environment

   iii. Severity

   - Mild [F1x.10, 562]: use when two or three symptoms are present
   - Moderate [F1x.20, 562]: use when four or five symptoms are present
   - Severe [F1x.20, 562]: use when six or more symptoms are present

c. Alternative: If a young person experiences problems associated with the use of stimulants that are not classifiable as stimulant use disorder, stimulant intoxication, stimulant withdrawal, stimulant intoxication delirium, stimulant withdrawal delirium, stimulant-induced neurocognitive disorder, stimulant-induced psychotic disorder, stimulant-induced bipolar disorder, stimulant-induced depressive disorder, stimulant-induced anxiety disorder, stimulant-induced sexual dysfunction, or stimulant-induced sleep disorder, consider unspecified stimulant-related disorder [F1x.99, 570].

20. Stimulant Intoxication [F1x.x2x, 567–569]

   a. Inclusion: Requires at least <u>two</u> of the following signs shortly after stimulant use.

    i. Tachycardia or bradycardia
    ii. Pupillary dilation
    iii. Elevated or lowered blood pressure
    iv. Perspiration or chills: *Over the last couple of hours, have you experienced chills or been sweating more than usual?*
    v. Nausea or vomiting: *Over the last couple of hours, have you felt sick to your stomach, felt nauseated, or even vomited?*
    vi. Evidence of weight loss
    vii. Psychomotor agitation or retardation
    viii. Muscular weakness, respiratory depression, chest pain, or cardiac arrhythmias
    ix. Confusion, seizures, dyskinesias, dystonias, or coma

b. Inclusion: Requires clinically significant problematic behavioral or psychological changes. *Since you began this episode of stimulant use, have you observed any significant changes in your mood, judgment, ability to interact with others, or sense of time? Have you engaged in problematic activities, or thought problematic thoughts, that you would not have without stimulants?*

c. Exclusion: If the symptoms are attributable to another medical condition or are better explained by another mental disorder, including intoxication with another substance, do not use this diagnosis.

d. Modifiers

    i. Specifiers

      • Specify the intoxicant: amphetamine, cocaine, or other stimulant
      • With perceptual disturbances [F1x.x29, 567]

21. Stimulant Withdrawal [F1x.23, 569–570]

a. Inclusion: Requires the following symptom, developing within hours to days of ceasing (or reducing) stimulant use that has been heavy or prolonged.

    i. Dysphoric mood: *Over the last few hours or days, have you felt much more down or depressed than usual?*

b. Inclusion: Also requires at least <u>two</u> of the following symptoms developing simultaneously.

i. Fatigue: *Over the last few hours or days, have you felt extremely sleepy or tired?*

ii. Vivid, unpleasant dreams: *Over the last few hours or days, have you experienced unusually vivid, unpleasant dreams?*

iii. Insomnia or hypersomnia: *Over the last few hours or days, have you found it more difficult than usual to get to sleep and to stay asleep? Alternatively, have you found that you have been sleeping much more than usual?*

iv. Increased appetite: *Over the last few hours or days, have you desired food much more than usual?*

v. Psychomotor retardation or agitation

c. Exclusion: If the symptoms are attributable to another medical condition or are better explained by another mental disorder, including intoxication with or withdrawal from another substance, do not use this diagnosis.

d. Modifiers

    i. Specifiers

        • Specify the intoxicant: amphetamine, cocaine, or other stimulant

22. Tobacco Use Disorder [xxx.x, 571–574]

a. Inclusion: Requires a problematic pattern of tobacco use leading to clinically significant impairment or distress as manifested by at least <u>two</u> of the following in a 12-month period.

i. Using more tobacco over a longer period than intended: *When you use tobacco, do you find that you use more, and for a longer time, than you planned to?*

ii. Persistent desire or unsuccessful effort to reduce tobacco use: *Do you want to cut back or stop using tobacco? Have you ever tried and failed to cut back or stop using tobacco?*

iii. Great deal of time spent: *Do you spend a great deal of your time obtaining tobacco, using tobacco, or recovering from your tobacco use?*

iv. Cravings: *Do you experience strong desires or cravings to use tobacco?*

v. Failure to fulfill major role obligations: *Have you repeatedly failed to fulfill major obligations at home, school, or work because of your tobacco use?*

vi. Continued use despite awareness of interpersonal or social problems: *Do you use tobacco even though you suspect, or even know, that your use creates or worsens interpersonal or social problems?*

vii. Giving up activities for tobacco: *Are there important social, occupational, or recreational activities that you have given up or reduced because of your tobacco use?*

viii. Use in hazardous situations: *Have you repeatedly used tobacco in situations in which it was physically hazardous, such as smoking in bed?*

ix. Continued use despite awareness of physical or psychological problems: *Do you use tobacco even though you suspect, or even know, that it creates or worsens problems with your mind and body?*

x. Tolerance as manifested by <u>either</u> of the following.

- Markedly increased amounts: *Do you find that in order to get the desired effect of tobacco, you need to consume much more than you used to?*
- Markedly diminished effects: *If you use the same amount of tobacco as you used to, do you find that it has a lot less effect on you than it used to?*

xi. Withdrawal as manifested by <u>either</u> of the following.

- Characteristic tobacco withdrawal syndrome: *When you stop using tobacco, do you undergo withdrawal?*
- The same substance is taken to relieve or avoid withdrawal symptoms: *Have you ever used tobacco to avoid or relieve symptoms of tobacco withdrawal?*

b. Modifiers

i. Specifiers

- In early remission
- In sustained remission
- On maintenance therapy
- In a controlled environment

ii. Severity

- Mild [Z72.0, 572]: use when two or three symptoms are present
- Moderate [F17.200, 572]: use when four or five symptoms are present
- Severe [F17.200, 572]: use when six or more symptoms are present

c. Alternatives: If a young person experiences clinically significant problems associated with the use of tobacco that do not meet criteria for a specific diagnosis, consider unspecified tobacco-related disorder [F17.209, 577].

23. Tobacco Withdrawal [F17.203, 575–576]

a. Inclusion: Requires at least <u>four</u> of the following symptoms developing within 24 hours of ceasing (or reducing) tobacco use that has been daily for at least several weeks.

i. Irritability, frustration, or anger: *Over the last 24 hours, have you felt more irritable, frustrated, or angry than usual?*

ii. Anxiety: *Over the last 24 hours, have you felt more worried or anxious than usual?*

iii. Difficulty concentrating: *Over the last 24 hours, have you had difficulty staying focused on a task or an activity?*

iv. Increased appetite: *Over the last 24 hours, have you desired food more than usual?*

v. Restlessness: *Over the last 24 hours, have you felt less able to remain at rest than usual?*

vi. Depressed mood: *Over the last 24 hours, have you been feeling more down or depressed than usual?*

vii. Insomnia: *Over the last 24 hours, have you found it more difficult than usual to get to sleep and to stay asleep?*

b. Exclusion: If the symptoms are attributable to another medical condition or are better explained by another mental disorder, including intoxication with or withdrawal from another substance, do not use this diagnosis.

24. Other (or Unknown) Substance Use Disorder [F19.x0, 577–580]

a. Inclusion: Requires a problematic pattern of use of an intoxicating substance not able to be classified within the other substance categories listed earlier, leading to clinically significant impairment or distress as manifested by at least <u>two</u> of the following in a 12-month period.

i. Taking more of the substance over a longer period than intended: *When you use the substance, do you find that you use it more often, or for a longer time, than you planned to?*

ii. Persistent desire or unsuccessful effort to reduce substance use: *Do you want to cut back or stop using the substance? Have you ever tried and failed to cut back or stop using the substance?*

iii. Great deal of time spent: *Do you spend a great deal of your time obtaining or using the substance or recovering from your substance use?*

iv. Cravings: *Do you experience strong desires or cravings to use the substance?*

v. Failure to fulfill major role obligations: *Have you repeatedly failed to fulfill major obligations at home, school, or work because of your substance use?*

vi. Continued use despite awareness of interpersonal or social problems: *Do you use the substance even though you suspect, or even know, that it creates or worsens interpersonal or social problems?*

vii. Giving up activities for the substance: *Are there important social, occupational, or recreational activities that you have given up or reduced because of your substance use?*

viii. Use in hazardous situations: *Have you repeatedly used the substance in situations in which it was physically hazardous, such as driving a car or operating a machine while intoxicated?*

ix. Continued use despite awareness of physical or psychological problems: *Do you use the substance even though you suspect, or even know, that it creates or worsens problems with your mind and body?*

x. Tolerance as manifested by <u>either</u> of the following.

- Markedly increased amounts: *Do you find that in order to get intoxicated or achieve the desired effect of substance use, you need to consume much more of the substance than you used to?*
- Markedly diminished effects: *If you use the same amount of the substance as you used to, do you find that it has a lot less effect on you than it used to?*

xi. Withdrawal as manifested by <u>either</u> of the following.

- Characteristic withdrawal syndrome for the substance: *When you stop using the substance, do you undergo withdrawal?*
- The same or a closely related substance is taken to relieve or avoid withdrawal symptoms: *Have*

you ever taken the substance or another substance to prevent withdrawal?

b. Modifiers

  i. Specifiers

  - In early remission
  - In sustained remission
  - In a controlled environment

  ii. Severity

  - Mild [F19.10, 578]: use when two or three symptoms are present
  - Moderate [F19.20, 578]: use when four or five symptoms are present
  - Severe [F19.20, 578]: use when six or more symptoms are present

25. Other (or Unknown) Substance Intoxication [F19.x29, 581–582]

  a. Inclusion: Development of a reversible substance-specific syndrome attributable to recent ingestion of (or exposure to) a substance that is not listed elsewhere or is unknown.

  b. Inclusion: Requires clinically significant problematic behavioral or psychological changes. *Since you began using this substance, have you observed any significant changes in your mood, judgment, ability to interact with others, or sense of time? Have you engaged in problematic activities, or thought problematic thoughts, that you would not have without using this substance?*

  c. Exclusion: If the symptoms are attributable to another medical condition or are better explained by another mental disorder, including intoxication with another substance, do not use this diagnosis.

26. Other (or Unknown) Substance Withdrawal [F19.239, 583–584]

  a. Inclusion: Development of a substance-specific syndrome shortly after the cessation of (or reduction in) use of the substance that has been heavy and prolonged.

  b. Inclusion: Requires clinically significant distress or impairment in social, occupational, or other important areas of functioning.

  c. Exclusion: If the symptoms are attributable to another medical condition or are better explained by another mental disorder, including withdrawal from another substance, do not use this diagnosis.

27. Gambling Disorder [F63.0, 585–589]

a. Inclusion: Requires persistent, recurrent problematic gambling that leads to clinically significant impairment or distress, lasting at least 12 months, as indicated by at least <u>four</u> of the following symptoms.

   i. Escalates spending on gambling: *Do you find that it takes increasing amounts of money to get the excitement you want from gambling?*

   ii. Is irritable when quitting: *When you try to reduce or quit gambling, are you irritable or restless?*

   iii. Is unable to quit: *Have you unsuccessfully tried to reduce or quit gambling on several occasions?*

   iv. Is preoccupied: *Are you preoccupied with gambling?*

   v. Gambles when distressed: *When you are feeling anxious, down, or helpless, do you gamble?*

   vi. Chases losses: *After you lose money, do you return another day to try to get even?*

   vii. Lies: *Do you lie to conceal how much you gamble?*

   viii. Loses relationships: *Have you lost a relationship, job, or opportunity because of your gambling?*

   ix. Borrows money: *Do you have to rely on other people for money to cover desperate financial situations caused by gambling?*

b. Exclusion: If the gambling behavior is better accounted for by a manic episode, do not use this diagnosis.

c. Modifiers

   i. Course

   • Episodic: Meeting diagnostic criteria at more than one time point, with symptoms subsiding between periods of gambling disorder for at least several months

   • Persistent: Experiencing continuous symptoms to meet diagnostic criteria for multiple years

   • In early remission

   • In sustained remission

   ii. Severity

   • Mild: use when four or five symptoms are present

- Moderate: use when six or seven symptoms are present
- Severe: use when eight or nine symptoms are present

Other Conditions That May Be a Focus of Clinical Attention

DSM-5 pp. 715–727

DSM-5 includes other conditions and problems that may be a focus of clinical attention or that may otherwise affect the diagnosis, course, prognosis, or treatment of a patient's mental disorder. These conditions and problems include, but are not limited to, the psychosocial and environmental problems that were coded on Axis IV in DSM-IV-TR (American Psychiatric Association 2000). The authors of DSM-5 provide a selected list of conditions and problems drawn from ICD-10-CM (usually Z codes). A condition or problem listed in the ICD-10 Z codes listed in Chapter 11, "Rating Scales and Alternative Diagnostic Systems," Table 11–3, may be coded if it is a reason for the current visit or helps to explain the need for a test, procedure, or treatment.

Conditions and problems from this list also may be included in the medical record as useful information on circumstances that may affect the patient's care, regardless of their relevance to the current visit. The conditions and problems listed in this section are not mental disorders. Their inclusion in DSM-5 is meant to draw attention to the scope of additional issues that are encountered in routine clinical practice and to provide a systematic listing that may be useful to clinicians in documenting these issues.

We include some commonly used codes in Chapter 11, "Rating Scales and Alternative Diagnostic Systems."

Chapter 7

A Brief Version of DSM-5

TABLE 7–1. Abbreviated DSM-5 criteria for common diagnoses

Diagnosis	Criteria/time	Symptoms
Neurodevelopmental disorders		
Attention-deficit/ hyperactivity disorder	≥6 for ≥6 months *OR*	Inattention: makes careless mistakes; cannot sustain attention; does not seem to listen; often does not follow through; struggles to organize tasks; dislikes mental effort; loses objects necessary for tasks; distractible; forgetful
	≥6 for ≥6 months	Hyperactivity/impulsivity: fidgets; leaves seat; runs or climbs; unable to remain quiet; on the go as if driven by a motor; talks excessively; blurts out answers; cannot wait turn; interrupts or intrudes without thinking
Intellectual disability	Both beginning in early childhood	Deficits in intellectual functions confirmed by standardized intelligence testing; deficits in adaptive functioning
Autism spectrum disorder	All 3 beginning in early childhood *AND*	Deficits in social-emotional reciprocity; deficits in nonverbal communicative behaviors; deficits in developing and maintaining relationships
	≥2	Stereotyped or repetitive speech, motor movements, or use of objects; excessive adherence to routines or excessive resistance to change; restricted interests of abnormal intensity or focus; hyperreactivity or hyporeactivity to sensory input

TABLE 7–1. Abbreviated DSM-5 criteria for common diagnoses (*continued*)

Diagnosis	Criteria/time	Symptoms
Neurodevelopmental disorders (*continued*)		
Specific learning disorder	≥1 for ≥6 months beginning during childhood *DESPITE* interventions to reduce difficulties	Inaccurate word reading; impaired reading comprehension; spelling difficulties; difficulties with written expression; difficulties with numbers; difficulties with mathematical reasoning
Schizophrenia spectrum and other psychotic disorders		
Schizophrenia	≥2 for ≥1 month *AND*	Delusions; hallucinations; disorganized speech; grossly disorganized or catatonic behavior; negative symptoms (at least one symptom must be delusions, hallucinations, or disorganized speech)
	≥6 months	Continuous signs of disturbance
Schizoaffective disorder	≥50% of the time *AND*	All criteria for schizophrenia
		Also experiences major depressive or manic episodes
	≥2 weeks	Delusions or hallucinations without depressive or manic episodes

TABLE 7-1. Abbreviated DSM-5 criteria for common diagnoses (*continued*)

Diagnosis	Criteria/time	Symptoms
Bipolar and related disorders		
Bipolar I disorder	Both for ≥1 week (or any duration if hospitalized) *AND*	Persistently elevated or irritable mood; persistently increased energy or activity
	≥3	Mania: inflated self-esteem or grandiosity; decreased need for sleep; pressured speech; racing thoughts; distractibility; risky behavior
Bipolar II disorder	≥3 for ≥4 days	Hypomania: inflated self-esteem or grandiosity; decreased need for sleep; pressured speech; racing thoughts; distractibility; increased goal-directed activity; risky behavior *without* psychosis or hospitalization
Depressive disorders		
Disruptive mood dysregulation disorder	≥3 outbursts per week for ≥12 months	Severe recurrent temper outbursts manifested verbally and/or behaviorally that are out of proportion to the situation and inconsistent with developmental level (diagnosis cannot be made in children younger than 6 years)
		Mood between outbursts is persistently irritable or angry

TABLE 7–1. Abbreviated DSM-5 criteria for common diagnoses (*continued*)

Diagnosis	Criteria/time	Symptoms
Depressive disorders (*continued*)		
Major depressive disorder	≥1 for ≥2 weeks *AND* ≥4 for ≥2 weeks	Depressed mood; loss of interest in activities or pleasure (anhedonia) Weight loss or decreased appetite; insomnia or hypersomnia; agitation or retardation; fatigue or loss of energy; excessive guilt; decreased ability to concentrate; thoughts of death or suicide
Anxiety disorders		
Separation anxiety disorder	≥3 for ≥4 weeks	Excessive distress with separation from home or caregivers; persistent worry about harm to caregivers; excessive worry about untoward event separating from caregiver; excessive reluctance to be alone; persistent reluctance to sleep away from home; repetitive nightmares about separation; repeated physical symptoms when separating
Panic disorder	≥4 *AND* ≥1 month	Palpitations; sweating; trembling; shortness of breath; choking; chest pain; nausea; dizziness; chills; paresthesias; derealization; fear of insanity; fear of death Persistent concern or worry about attacks; significant behavior change related to attacks

TABLE 7–1. Abbreviated DSM-5 criteria for common diagnoses (*continued*)

Diagnosis	Criteria/time	Symptoms
Anxiety disorders (*continued*)		
Generalized anxiety disorder	≥3 for ≥6 months	Restlessness; easy fatigability; difficulty concentrating; irritability; muscle tension; sleep disturbance; avoidance of situations
Obsessive-compulsive and related disorders		
Obsessive-compulsive disorder	≥1 hour/day	Obsessions: recurrent and intrusive thoughts, urges, images that a person attempts to ignore or suppress through compulsive acts *AND/OR*
		Compulsions: repetitive behaviors or mental acts to reduce distress
Trauma- and stressor-related disorders		
Reactive attachment disorder	Both beginning before 5 years old	Experience of extreme insufficient care
		Consistent pattern of emotionally withdrawn behavior toward caregivers; persistent social and emotional disturbance

TABLE 7–1. Abbreviated DSM-5 criteria for common diagnoses *(continued)*

Diagnosis	Criteria/time	Symptoms
Trauma- and stressor-related disorders *(continued)*		
Posttraumatic stress disorder (6 years or younger)	≥1 for ≥1 month *AND*	Intrusive experiences: distressing memories; dreams; flashbacks; reminder exposure distress; physiological reactions
	≥2 for ≥1 month *AND*	Arousal: irritability and angry outbursts; hypervigilance; exaggerated startle; impaired concentration; sleep disturbance
	≥1 for ≥1 month *OR*	Avoidance of: internal reminders; external reminders
	≥2 for ≥1 month	Negative cognitions: negative emotional states; diminished interest in significant activities; socially withdrawn; reduced expression of positive emotions

TABLE 7–1. Abbreviated DSM-5 criteria for common diagnoses *(continued)*

Diagnosis	Criteria/time	Symptoms
Trauma- and stressor-related disorders *(continued)*		
Posttraumatic stress disorder (older than 6 years)	≥1 for ≥1 month *AND*	Intrusive experiences: distressing memories; dreams; flashbacks; reminder exposure distress; physiological reactions
	≥1 for ≥1 month *AND*	Avoidance of: internal reminders; external reminders
	≥2 for ≥1 month *AND*	Negative cognitions: impaired memories; negative self-image; blame; negative emotional states; decreased participation; detachment; inability to experience pleasure
	≥2 for ≥1 month	Arousal: irritability and angry outbursts; recklessness; hypervigilance; exaggerated startle; impaired concentration; sleep disturbance

TABLE 7–1. Abbreviated DSM-5 criteria for common diagnoses (*continued*)

Diagnosis	Criteria/time	Symptoms
Feeding and eating disorders		
Pica	≥1 month	Persistent consumption of nonnutritive, nonfood substances that is inconsistent with developmental stage and cultural practices
Anorexia nervosa	All 3	Persistent energy intake restriction; intense fear of gaining weight or persistent behavior that interferes with weight gain; disturbance in self-perceived body shape or weight
Bulimia nervosa	Both at least weekly for ≥3 months	Recurrent episodes of binge eating; self-evaluation unduly influenced by body shape and weight
		Recurrent inappropriate compensatory behaviors to prevent weight gain
Elimination disorders		
Enuresis (≥5 years)	≥2 times weekly for ≥3 months	Repeated passage of urine into bed or clothes not attributable to a substance or another medical condition
Encopresis (≥4 years)	≥1 monthly for ≥3 months	Repeated passage of feces into inappropriate places not attributable to a substance or another medical condition

TABLE 7–1. Abbreviated DSM-5 criteria for common diagnoses *(continued)*

Diagnosis	Criteria/time	Symptoms
Disruptive, impulse-control, and conduct disorders		
Oppositional defiant disorder	≥4 for ≥6 months; if younger than 5 years, symptoms on most days; if older than 5 years, symptoms at least weekly	Often loses temper; often touchy or easily annoyed; often angry and resentful; often argues with adults; often defies rules or authority figures; often annoys others; often blames others; spiteful or vindictive
Intermittent explosive disorder	≥1 in a person ≥6 years	Recurrent, impulsive (or anger-based) verbal outbursts ≥2 times weekly for ≥3 months; ≥3 impulsive (or anger-based) behavioral outbursts resulting in property damage or injury to animals or persons in a 12-month period

TABLE 7–1. Abbreviated DSM-5 criteria for common diagnoses *(continued)*

Diagnosis	Criteria/time	Symptoms
Disruptive, impulse-control, and conduct disorders *(continued)*		
Conduct disorder	≥3 in the past 12 months *AND* ≥1 in the past 6 months	Often bullies or threatens others; often initiates physical fights; uses a weapon; physically cruel to people; physically cruel to animals; stealing while confronting a victim; forcing someone into sexual activity; deliberately sets fire to cause damage; deliberately destroys property; breaks into someone else's dwelling or car; frequently lies to obtain favors or avoid obligations; steals items of nontrivial value; stays out at night without permission; runs away from home overnight; often truant from school

Source. American Psychiatric Association 2013.

SECTION III

Additional Tools and Clinical Guidance

Chapter 8

A Stepwise Approach to Differential Diagnosis

Although diagnoses are the known result of an interview, a good interviewer should generate more hypotheses than diagnoses because an interviewer is investigating the nature of a person's distress (Feinstein 1967). In these investigations, the set of possibilities is large. Although an entire manual has been designed specifically to teach the differential diagnosis for DSM-5 (First 2014), it is helpful to review the following general seven-step approach to generating the differential diagnosis in children and adolescents. As you develop your clinical decision making, it is helpful to follow these steps sequentially so that you will consider each possible cause of mental distress.

Step 1: Consider to What Extent the Signs and Symptoms Are Intentionally Produced

Always consider if a patient is intentionally producing findings, because an honest report of psychiatric symptoms and signs is the true foundation for developing a diagnosis and treatment plan. An honest report strengthens the therapeutic alliance, whereas a dishonest report weakens the therapeutic alliance.

If intentionally produced findings are associated with an obvious external award—such as time off from school or work or change in caregivers—consider the possibility of malingering. Remember that malingering can be concomitant with other medical and psychiatric diagnoses.

If intentionally produced findings are associated with the desire to be perceived as ill or impaired, consider factitious disorder.

A patient can also unconsciously produce signs or symptoms to resolve a conflict, to validate his inability to function, or to attempt to secure assistance. In these situations, consider one of the somatic symptom and related disorders.

Step 2: Consider to What Extent the Signs and Symptoms Are Related to a Developmental Conflict or Stage

If you are thoroughly evaluating a young child, your evaluation should eventually include formal developmental assessment, a skill beyond the scope of this book. Even when you are interviewing older children, adolescents, and adults, however, you should consider a patient's developmental stage, which can be quite different from the developmental stage you would expect based on his age, background, and education (summarized in Chapter 12, "Developmental Milestones"). A thorough social history also will give you a sense of how a patient's current behavior relates to his usual behavior. Even in a brief interview, it is useful to observe how your patient communicates and behaves and compare his communication and behavior with those appropriate for his age, culture, and education. If you observe a disjunction, consider these possibilities:

- The patient is experiencing a transient regression in response to a particular event.
- The patient is using an immature defense mechanism, which may indicate a personality trait or disorder.
- The patient is experiencing a developmental conflict in a particular relationship.
- The patient has a developmental delay or intellectual impairment.

Step 3: Consider to What Extent the Signs and Symptoms Are Related to a Caregiver Conflict

Human beings are, in the words of the philosopher Alasdair MacIntyre, "dependent rational animals" because we depend on "particular others for protection and sustenance" (MacIntyre 2012, p. 1). This dependence is acute for children and adolescents. By degrees of ability, age, development, impairment, and temperament, children and adolescents depend on both adults and fellow children as caregivers. Caregivers can aid or injure a child or an adolescent. As you evaluate a child or an adolescent, observe how he does (or does not) speak about the caregivers in his life, either directly or through transitional objects. As you observe, consider these possibilities:

- A caregiver and the patient have communication difficulties or cultural differences.
- A caregiver is a poor fit with the patient.
- A caregiver is abusing, neglecting, or otherwise harming the patient.

Step 4: Consider to What Extent the Signs and Symptoms Are Related to Substances

The variety of substances that people use and misuse is remarkable, as are the clinical effects of substance use. People can experience mental distress during substance use, intoxication, and withdrawal. When you seek the cause of a patient's distress, always consider drugs of abuse, as well as prescription, over-the-counter, and herbal medicines. Ask about substances ingested both intentionally and unintentionally. People often underreport their use of substances, so consider these possibilities:

- Substances directly cause the patient's psychiatric signs and symptoms, a substance/medication-induced mental disorder.
- A patient uses substances because of a mental disorder and its sequelae.
- A patient uses substances and experiences psychiatric signs and symptoms, but the substance use and signs and symptoms are unrelated.

Step 5: Consider to What Extent the Signs and Symptoms Are Related to Another Medical Condition

A patient can present with another medical condition that mimics psychiatric signs and symptoms. Sometimes, his presentation with these findings is a sentinel event that occurs in advance of the other stigmata of a medical condition. Alternatively, he may develop psychiatric signs and symptoms years after his presentation for another medical condition. Clues that another medical condition may be related to a mental disorder include an atypical presentation, abnormal age at onset, and abnormal course. Consider these possibilities:

- Another medical condition directly alters the patient's psychiatric signs and symptoms.
- Another medical condition indirectly alters the patient's psychiatric signs and symptoms, as through a psychological mechanism.
- The treatment for another medical condition directly alters the patient's psychiatric signs and symptoms.
- The patient's mental disorder, or its treatment, causes or exacerbates another medical condition.
- The patient has a mental disorder and another medical condition, but they are causally unrelated.

Step 6: Consider to What Extent the Signs and Symptoms Are Related to a Mental Disorder

"Normality" covers a wide range of behaviors and thoughts that vary across cultural groups and developmental stages. In DSM-5, a mental disorder causes a "clinically significant disturbance in an individual's cognition, emotional regulation, or behavior that reflects a dysfunction in the psychological, biological, or developmental processes underlying mental functioning" (American Psychiatric Association 2013, p. 20). Diagnoses are summaries of information that allow you to categorize the experiences of a distressed person in a way that generates useful information about prognosis, preferred treatment strategies, and expected outcomes. DSM-5 seeks parsimony, but diagnoses are not mutually exclusive, so consider these possibilities:

- Condition A predisposes a patient to Condition B, or vice versa.
- An underlying condition, such as a genetic predisposition, predisposes a patient to both Conditions A and B.

- A mediating factor, such as alterations in reward systems, influences a patient's susceptibility to both Conditions A and B.
- Conditions A and B may be part of a more complex and unified syndrome that has been artificially split in the diagnostic system.
- The relation between Conditions A and B is artificially enhanced by overlaps in the diagnostic criteria.
- The comorbidity between Conditions A and B is coincidental.

Step 7: Consider Whether No Mental Disorder Is Present

When a patient's symptoms and presentation do not fulfill the criteria for a specific mental disorder but cause clinically significant distress or impairment, consider alternatives. If the distress or impairment has developed as a maladaptive response to an identifiable psychosocial stressor, consider an adjustment disorder. If the patient's symptoms are not secondary to a stressor, consider an other specified diagnosis (when you are specifying why a patient's experience does not meet the criteria for a specific diagnosis) or an unspecified diagnosis (when you do not specify why a patient's experience does not meet the criteria for a specific diagnosis) or the possibility of no psychiatric diagnosis at all. After all, the boundaries between normality and abnormality are ultimately determined through the exercise of experienced judgment.

Chapter 9

The Mental Status Examination: A Psychiatric Glossary

Just as a physical examination commonly moves from head to toe, the mental status examination begins with a child or an adolescent's outer appearance and progressively proceeds into her interior life. To describe these experiences, clinicians use a specialized language. Comprehensive glossaries of psychiatric terms are available elsewhere (Shahrokh et al. 2011). The following list includes both brief definitions of some of the more specialized terms used in the mental status examination and a way to organize your findings.

Mental Status Examination

Appearance

Note a person's dress, cleanliness, habitus, posture, appropriateness of her appearance for her age, and ability to form and maintain eye contact.

Behavior

Describe any mannerisms (unnecessary behaviors that are a part of goal-directed behavior), stereotypies (non-goal-directed behavior), tics (involuntary, recurrent, nonrhythmic movement or vocalization), posturing (striking a pose and maintaining it), presence of waxy flexibility (resistance of limbs to passive motion), catalepsy (maintaining of any position), tremor, agitation, movement retardation, or signs of extrapyramidal symptoms or tardive dyskinesia. Comment on the person's ability to relate socially during your encounter.

Speech

Describe the rate, tone, rhythm, volume, general quality, and presence of any latency (a pause of several seconds before responding to a question).

Emotion

Describe the quality, type, stability, range, intensity, and appropriateness of a person's emotional state. Describe the person's mood, sustained emotional state, and affect (i.e., the observable behaviors that are expressions of emotion).

Thought Process

Describe how a person thinks, and note any evidence of the loosening of her associations—ranging from intact, circumstantial (providing unnecessary details but eventually answering a question), tangential (only touching on your question before heading in a different direction), loose (providing responses unrelated to a question), flight of ideas (forming an illogical group of associations), to word salad (randomly using words). Also observe for distractibility (being easily diverted by extraneous stimuli), derailment (running ideas into each other), perseveration, verbigeration (prolonged repetition of isolated words), echolalia (repetition of words or statements of others), neologisms (creation of words), clang association (words chosen purely for sound), alliteration, pressured speech (increased, rapid speech that is often loud and difficult to interrupt), decreased latency of response (answering questions before you can finish asking them), increased latency of response, poverty of speech, blocking (sudden stops in the middle of a thought sequence), mutism (absence of speech), and aphonia (ability to only whisper or croak).

Thought Content

Comment on what a person discusses, including the presence of ideation, intent, or plans to harm self or others; phobias (intense, unreasonable fears); obsessions (idea, image, or desire that dominates thought); compulsions (irresistible impulse to perform an action); hallucinations (the perception of an absent stimulus); illusions (misperception of an actual stimulus); delusions (fixed, firm, false beliefs that are not a part of person's culture or religion); persecution; paranoia; guilt; passivity; and ideas of reference (perceptions that unrelated stimuli refer directly to the person).

Cognition and Intellectual Resources

Observe a person's orientation, recent and remote memory, ability to calculate, and ability to abstract and to interpret proverbs. Comment on the person's ability to control impulses during the interview. When known, comment on the person's IQ and learning style.

Judgment and Insight

Observe and comment on the person's level of insight into her own difficulties, especially if she denies or appreciates her problems. Judgment within a mental status examination refers to the appropriateness of a person's decision making as related to both her presenting condition and her developmental age.

Chapter 10

Selected DSM-5
Assessment Measures

Contrary to popular characterizations of the DSM texts
as fixed as scripture, the authors of DSM-5 (American Psychiatric Association 2013) describe the manual as subject to constant revision, with plans to update the manual as the science
demands. This commitment reaffirms the ways that DSM is a
pragmatic text for current clinical use (Kinghorn 2011). DSM-
5's pragmatism extends to planning for its eventual succes-
sors. In Section III, "Emerging Measures and Models," the
authors of DSM-5 include several assessment tools, rating
scales, and alternative diagnoses. Taken together, these constitute both valuable tools for current use and possible ways
forward for DSM as a diagnostic system.

At present, the main text of DSM-5 preserves the categorical model of mental illness. The categorical model, in which
a person does or does not have a mental illness on the basis
of the presence or absence of symptoms, was first introduced
in DSM-III and is widely recognized for its ability to hold together the various practitioners and researchers who care for
and study persons with mental illness (American Psychiatric
Association 1980).

The great achievement of the categorical model has been
diagnostic reliability (i.e., the ability of different practitioners
to agree on the same diagnosis for a particular person). One
shortcoming of the categorical model has been limited diagnostic validity (i.e., the ability of practitioners to make an accurate diagnosis) (Kendell and Jablensky 2003).

In various ways, each of the tools in Section III of DSM-5
attempts to improve the reliability and validity of psychiatric
diagnoses. These tools are diverse, but we find that all of
these measures are ways that practitioners can personalize
the diagnostic criteria for particular patients.

In this chapter, we introduce several of these measures as
aids to clinical practice with children and adolescents.

Level 1 and 2 Cross-Cutting Symptom Measures

Most young people will first seek help for mental distress from someone they already know. Within medicine, this is usually a physician, nurse, school counselor, or other professional whose principal role or specialty is not the provision of mental health services. Indeed, most mental health care occurs in the offices of primary care practitioners. To address the gap between the mental health training that these practitioners possess and the volume of mental health care they provide, DSM-5 provides screening tools for use in either primary care or mental health settings. These brief, easy-to-read, paper-based tools can be completed before a clinical encounter by the patient or someone who knows him well. The tools are available in this chapter, in Section III of DSM-5, and online at www.psychiatry.org/dsm5. They can be reproduced and used, without additional permission, for clinical and research evaluations.

Each tool has a series of short questions about recent symptoms; for example, "During the past two (2) weeks, how much (or how often) has your child seemed angry or lost his/her temper?" These screening questions assess core symptoms for the major diagnoses. For each symptom statement, a patient or his caregiver will assess how much this bothered him with a five-point scale: none (0), slight (1), mild (2), moderate (3), or severe (4). Each tool is designed to be easily scored. If a patient reports a clinically significant problem in any domain, you should consider a more detailed assessment tool; in this example, that would be a tool for assessing anger.

DSM-5 includes a hierarchy of screening tools. The initial assessment, described in the previous paragraph, is the Level 1 Cross-Cutting Symptom Measure, which is completed before an initial evaluation by the person seeking assessment or by the caregiver of a child or an adolescent. The version for children ages 6–17 (there is no version for children younger than 6) includes 25 questions assessing 12 domains and is available in a format for a child or an adolescent to complete on his or her own or for a caregiver to complete. For most, but not all, of the symptom domains screened for in the Level 1 Cross-Cutting Symptom Measure, separate Level 2 Cross-Cutting Symptom Measures are available for specific areas of concern, including anger, anxiety, depression, inattention, mania, repetitive thoughts and behaviors, sleep disturbance, somatic symptom, and substance use.

When Level 1 and 2 assessments are used, they can help a practitioner identify and characterize the presenting problems. But they have another potential benefit after the initial assessment: to help measure treatment response and progress toward recovery. DSM-5 suggests using the Level 2 Cross-Cutting Symptom Measures at your first evaluation of a patient in part so that you can establish a baseline and then revisit that assessment periodically to assess progress. These measures assess dimensions rather than diagnoses, which means they are not designed to tell you the degree of likelihood of identifying a specific diagnosis. Their strength is that they allow you to track different symptom domains, such as the depressive symptoms of a patient with schizophrenia in addition to his psychotic symptoms.

Systematic use of these cross-cutting assessments will alert you to significant changes in a patient's symptomatology and will provide measurable outcomes for treatment plans. They also may alert researchers to lacunae in the current diagnostic system.

For your convenience, Figures 10–1 and 10–2 include the child- and caregiver-rated versions of the Level 1 tool.

Practitioners using the Level 1 tools are encouraged to further explore reports of even seemingly slight problems with inattention, psychosis, substance use, and suicidal ideation or attempts. For the other domains, practitioners are encouraged to explore symptoms identified at the next, higher level of severity (mild or several days) or greater. The Level 2 measures are easily accessed online at www.psychiatry.org/practice/dsm/dsm5/online-assessment-measures. The suggested Level 2 measures are described in Table 10–1.

Cultural Formulation Interview

Another way the authors of DSM-5 are seeking to improve the diagnostic system is by attending to the cultural specificity of mental distress and illness. Asking about a patient's and caregiver's cultural understanding of sickness and health is an efficient way to build a therapeutic alliance while gathering pertinent information (Lim 2015). In addition, performing a cultural assessment personalizes the diagnosis, which increases its accuracy (Bäärnhielm and Scarpinati

Name: _____ Age: _____ Sex: ☐ Male ☐ Female Date: _____

Instructions: The questions below ask about things that might have bothered you. For each question, circle the number that best describes how much (or how often) you have been bothered by each problem during the **past TWO (2) WEEKS.**

	During the past **TWO (2) WEEKS,** how much (or how often) have you...	None Not at all	Slight Rare, less than a day or two	Mild Several days	Moderate More than half the days	Severe Nearly every day	Highest Domain Score (clinician)
I.	1.	Been bothered by stomachaches, headaches, or other aches and pains?	0	1	2	3	4	
	2.	Worried about your health or about getting sick?	0	1	2	3	4	
II.	3.	Been bothered by not being able to fall asleep or stay asleep, or by waking up too early?	0	1	2	3	4	
III.	4.	Been bothered by not being able to pay attention when you were in class or doing homework or reading a book or playing a game?	0	1	2	3	4	
IV.	5.	Had less fun doing things than you used to?	0	1	2	3	4	
	6.	Felt sad or depressed for several hours?	0	1	2	3	4	
V. &	7.	Felt more irritated or easily annoyed than usual?	0	1	2	3	4	
VI.	8.	Felt angry or lost your temper?	0	1	2	3	4	

FIGURE 10–1. DSM-5 Self-Rated Level 1 Cross-Cutting Symptom Measure—Child Age 11–17.

		None Not at all	Slight Rare, less than a day or two	Mild Several days	Moderate More than half the days	Severe Nearly every day	Highest Domain Score (clinician)
	During the past **TWO (2) WEEKS,** how much (or how often) have you...						
VII.	9. Started lots more projects than usual or done more risky things than usual?	0	1	2	3	4	
	10. Slept less than usual but still had a lot of energy?	0	1	2	3	4	
VIII.	11. Felt nervous, anxious, or scared?	0	1	2	3	4	
	12. Not been able to stop worrying?	0	1	2	3	4	
	13. Not been able to do things you wanted to or should have done, because they made you feel nervous?	0	1	2	3	4	
IX.	14. Heard voices—when there was no one there—speaking about you or telling you what to do or saying bad things to you?	0	1	2	3	4	
	15. Had visions when you were completely awake—that is, seen something or someone that no one else could see?	0	1	2	3	4	

FIGURE 10–1. DSM-5 Self-Rated Level 1 Cross-Cutting Symptom Measure—Child Age 11–17. (*continued*)

		None Not at all	Slight Rare, less than a day or two	Mild Several days	Moderate More than half the days	Severe Nearly every day	Highest Domain Score (clinician)
	During the past **TWO (2) WEEKS,** how much (or how often) have you...						
X.							
16.	Had thoughts that kept coming into your mind that you would do something bad or that something bad would happen to you or to someone else?	0	1	2	3	4	
17.	Felt the need to check on certain things over and over again, like whether a door was locked or whether the stove was turned off?	0	1	2	3	4	
18.	Worried a lot about things you touched being dirty or having germs or being poisoned?	0	1	2	3	4	
19.	Felt you had to do things in a certain way, like counting or saying special things, to keep something bad from happening?	0	1	2	3	4	

FIGURE 10–1. DSM-5 Self-Rated Level 1 Cross-Cutting Symptom Measure—Child Age 11–17. *(continued)*

	In the past **TWO (2) WEEKS,** have you...		
XI.	20.	Had an alcoholic beverage (beer, wine, liquor, etc.)?	☐ Yes	☐ No
	21.	Smoked a cigarette, a cigar, or pipe, or used snuff or chewing tobacco?	☐ Yes	☐ No
	22.	Used drugs like marijuana, cocaine or crack, club drugs (like Ecstasy), hallucinogens (like LSD), heroin, inhalants or solvents (like glue), or methamphetamine (like speed)?	☐ Yes	☐ No
	23.	Used any medicine without a doctor's prescription to get high or change the way you feel (e.g., painkillers [like Vicodin], stimulants [like Ritalin or Adderall], sedatives or tranquilizers [like sleeping pills or Valium], or steroids)?	☐ Yes	☐ No
XII.	24.	In the last 2 weeks, have you thought about killing yourself or committing suicide?	☐ Yes	☐ No
	25.	Have you EVER tried to kill yourself?	☐ Yes	☐ No

FIGURE 10–1.   DSM-5 Self-Rated Level 1 Cross-Cutting Symptom Measure—Child Age 11–17. *(continued)*

Child's Name: _____   Age: _____   Sex: ☐ Male ☐ Female   Date: _____

Relationship with the child: _____

Instructions *(to the parent or guardian of child)*: The questions below ask about things that might have bothered your child. For each question, circle the number that best describes how much (or how often) your child has been bothered by each problem during the past TWO (2) WEEKS.

	During the past **TWO (2) WEEKS,** how much (or how often) has your child...	None Not at all	Slight Rare, less than a day or two	Mild Several days	Moderate More than half the days	Severe Nearly every day	Highest Domain Score (clinician)
I.	1.	Complained of stomachaches, headaches, or other aches and pains?	0	1	2	3	4	
	2.	Said he/she was worried about his/her health or about getting sick?	0	1	2	3	4	
II.	3.	Had problems sleeping—that is, trouble falling asleep, staying asleep, or waking up too early?	0	1	2	3	4	
III.	4.	Had problems paying attention when he/she was in class or doing his/her homework or reading a book or playing a game?	0	1	2	3	4	
IV.	5.	Had less fun doing things than he/she used to?	0	1	2	3	4	
	6.	Seemed sad or depressed for several hours?	0	1	2	3	4	

FIGURE 10–2. DSM-5 Parent/Guardian-Rated Level 1 Cross-Cutting Symptom Measure—Child Age 6–17.

	During the past TWO (2) WEEKS, how much (or how often) has your child...	None Not at all	Slight Rare, less than a day or two	Mild Several days	Moderate More than half the days	Severe Nearly every day	Highest Domain Score (clinician)
V. &	7.	Seemed more irritated or easily annoyed than usual?	0	1	2	3	4	
VI.	8.	Seemed angry or lost his/her temper?	0	1	2	3	4	
VII.	9.	Started lots more projects than usual or did more risky things than usual?	0	1	2	3	4	
	10.	Slept less than usual for him/her, but still had lots of energy?	0	1	2	3	4	
VIII.	11.	Said he/she felt nervous, anxious, or scared?	0	1	2	3	4	
	12.	Not been able to stop worrying?	0	1	2	3	4	
	13.	Said he/she couldn't do things he/she wanted to or should have done, because they made him/her feel nervous?	0	1	2	3	4	
IX.	14.	Said that he/she heard voices—when there was no one there—speaking about him/her or telling him/her what to do or saying bad things to him/her?	0	1	2	3	4	
	15.	Said that he/she had a vision when he/she was completely awake—that is, saw something or someone that no one else could see?	0	1	2	3	4	

FIGURE 10–2. DSM-5 Parent/Guardian-Rated Level 1 Cross-Cutting Symptom Measure—Child Age 6–17. *(continued)*

During the past **TWO (2) WEEKS,** how much (or how often) has your child...	**None** Not at all	**Slight** Rare, less than a day or two	**Mild** Several days	**Moderate** More than half the days	**Severe** Nearly every day	**Highest Domain Score** (clinician)
X.						
16. Said that he/she had thoughts that kept coming into his/her mind that he/she would do something bad or that something bad would happen to him/her or to someone else?	0	1	2	3	4	
17. Said he/she felt the need to check on certain things over and over again, like whether a door was locked or whether the stove was turned off?	0	1	2	3	4	
18. Seemed to worry a lot about things he/she touched being dirty or having germs or being poisoned?	0	1	2	3	4	
19. Said that he/she had to do things in a certain way, like counting or saying special things out loud, in order to keep something bad from happening?	0	1	2	3	4	

FIGURE 10–2. DSM-5 Parent/Guardian-Rated Level 1 Cross-Cutting Symptom Measure—Child Age 6–17. *(continued)*

			Yes	No	
XI.		In the past **TWO (2) WEEKS**, has your child …			
	20.	Had an alcoholic beverage (beer, wine, liquor, etc.)?	☐ Yes	☐ No	☐ Don't Know
	21.	Smoked a cigarette, a cigar, or pipe, or used snuff or chewing tobacco?	☐ Yes	☐ No	☐ Don't Know
	22.	Used drugs like marijuana, cocaine or crack, club drugs (like ecstasy), hallucinogens (like LSD), heroin, inhalants or solvents (like glue), or methamphetamine (like speed)?	☐ Yes	☐ No	☐ Don't Know
	23.	Used any medicine without a doctor's prescription (e.g., painkillers [like Vicodin], stimulants [like Ritalin or Adderall], sedatives or tranquilizers [like sleeping pills or Valium], or steroids)?	☐ Yes	☐ No	☐ Don't Know
XII.	24.	In the past **TWO (2) WEEKS,** has he/she talked about wanting to kill himself/herself or about wanting to commit suicide?	☐ Yes	☐ No	☐ Don't Know
	25.	Has he/she EVER tried to kill himself/herself?	☐ Yes	☐ No	☐ Don't Know

FIGURE 10–2. DSM-5 Parent/Guardian-Rated Level 1 Cross-Cutting Symptom Measure—Child Age 6–17. *(continued)*

Selected DSM-5 Assessment Measures

TABLE 10–1. DSM-5 Self-Rated Level 1 Cross-Cutting Symptom Measure—Child Age 11–17: domains, thresholds for further inquiry, and associated Level 2 measures

Domain	Domain Name	Threshold to guide further inquiry	DSM-5 Level 2 Cross-Cutting Symptom Measure available online
I.	Somatic Symptoms	Mild or greater	LEVEL 2—Somatic Symptom—Child Age 11–17 (Patient Health Questionnaire Somatic Symptom Severity [PHQ-15])
II.	Sleep Problems	Mild or greater	LEVEL 2—Sleep Disturbance—Child Age 11–17 (PROMIS—Sleep Disturbance—Short Form)[a]
III.	Inattention	Slight or greater	None
IV.	Depression	Mild or greater	LEVEL 2—Depression—Child Age 11–17 (PROMIS Emotional Distress—Depression—Pediatric Item Bank)
V.	Anger	Mild or greater	LEVEL 2—Anger—Child Age 11–17 (PROMIS Emotional Distress—Calibrated Anger Measure—Pediatric)
VI.	Irritability	Mild or greater	LEVEL 2—Irritability—Child Age 11–17 (Affective Reactivity Index [ARI])
VII.	Mania	Mild or greater	LEVEL 2—Mania—Child Age 11–17 (Altman Self-Rating Mania Scale [ASRM])

TABLE 10–1. DSM-5 Self-Rated Level 1 Cross-Cutting Symptom Measure—Child Age 11–17: domains, thresholds for further inquiry, and associated Level 2 measures (continued)

Domain	Domain Name	Threshold to guide further inquiry	DSM-5 Level 2 Cross-Cutting Symptom Measure available online
VIII.	Anxiety	Mild or greater	LEVEL 2—Anxiety—Child Age 11–17 (PROMIS Emotional Distress—Anxiety—Pediatric Item Bank)
IX.	Psychosis	Slight or greater	None
X.	Repetitive Thoughts & Behaviors	Mild or greater	LEVEL 2—Repetitive Thoughts and Behaviors—Child 11–17 (adapted from the Children's Florida Obsessive-Compulsive Inventory [C-FOCI] Severity Scale)
XI.	Substance Use	Yes/Don't Know	LEVEL 2—Substance Use—Child Age 11–17 (adapted from the NIDA-modified ASSIST)
XII.	Suicidal Ideation/ Suicide Attempts	Yes/Don't Know	None

aNot validated for children by the PROMIS group but found to have acceptable test-retest reliability with child informants in the DSM-5 Field Trial.

Rosso 2009). In Section III of DSM-5, in "Cultural Formulation," the authors discuss cultural syndromes, cultural idioms of distress, and cultural explanations of perceived causes.

To use this cultural information in an interview, it is beneficial to first define a few terms. A *cultural syndrome* is a group of clustered psychiatric symptoms specific to a particular culture or community. The syndrome may or may not be recognized as an illness by members of a community or by observers. A classic example is *ataque de nervios,* a syndrome of mental distress characterized by the sudden onset of intense fear, often experienced physically as a sensation of heat rising in the chest, that may result in aggressive or suicidal behavior (Lewis-Fernández et al. 2015). The syndrome is often associated with familial distress in Latino communities (Lizardi et al. 2009). A *cultural idiom of distress* such as *ataque de nervios* is a way of discussing mental distress or suffering shared by members of a particular community. Finally, a *cultural explanation of perceived cause* provides an explanatory model of why mental distress or illness occurs (American Psychiatric Association 2013).

The Cultural Formulation Interview (CFI) is a structured tool, updated for DSM-5, to assess the influence of culture in a particular patient's experience of distress. You can use the CFI at any time during an interview, but the DSM-5 authors suggest using it when a patient is disengaged during an interview, when you are struggling to reach a diagnosis, or when you are laboring to assess the dimensional severity of a diagnosis (American Psychiatric Association 2013). Although use of the CFI has been studied mostly in immigrant communities (Martínez 2009), you should not limit its use to situations in which you perceive the patient as culturally different from yourself. You can use the CFI profitably in any setting because "cultural" accounts of why people get ill and why people return to health occur not only in immigrant communities but in all communities. A person who you believe shares your own cultural account of illness and health often has a very different understanding of why people become ill and how they can become well. Furthermore, the CFI is the most patient-centered portion of DSM-5, and using it particularizes the diagnostic process.

The CFI is not a scored system of symptoms but rather a series of prompts to help you assess how a patient understands his distress, its etiology, its treatment, and prognosis.

The CFI can be incorporated into a diagnostic examination when you want to personalize the diagnosis and build a therapeutic alliance. If you want to learn more about the CFI, you should review the materials in Section III of DSM-5 or the handbook published to teach the CFI (Lewis-Fernández et al. 2015). However, those versions of the CFI are mostly designed for adults. Here, we include an adapted version of the supplemental CFI questions specific to children and adolescents.

Suggested introduction to the child or adolescent: *We have talked about the concerns of your family. Now I would like to know more about how you feel about being ___ years old.*

Feelings of age appropriateness in different settings: *Do you feel you are like other people your age? In what way? Do you sometimes feel different from other people your age? In what way?*

If a child or an adolescent acknowledges sometimes feeling different: *Does this feeling of being different happen more at home, at school, at work, and/or some other place? Do you feel that your family is different from other families? Do you use different languages? With whom and when? Does your name have any special meaning for you? Your family? Your community? Is there something special about you that you like or that you are proud of?*

Age-related stressors and supports: *What do you like about being a person at home? At school? With friends? What don't you like about being a person at home? At school? With friends? Who is there to support you when you feel you need it? At home? At school? Among your friends?*

Age-related expectations: *What do your parents or grandparents expect from a person your age in terms of chores, schoolwork, play, or religious observance? What do your schoolteachers expect from a person your age?*

If a child or an adolescent has siblings: *What do your siblings expect from a person your age? What do other people your age expect from a person your age?*

Transition to adulthood/maturity (for adolescents only): *Are there any important celebrations or events in your community to recognize reaching a certain age or growing up? When is a youth considered ready to become an adult in your family or community? When is a youth considered ready to become an adult according to your schoolteachers? What is good or difficult about becoming a young woman or a young man in your family? In your school? In your community? How do you feel about "growing up" or becom-*

*ing an adult? In what ways are your life and responsibilities differ-
ent from the lives and responsibilities of your parents?*

**Suggested questions for the caregiver of a child or an ado-
lescent:** *Can you tell me about the child's particular place in the
family (e.g., oldest boy, only girl)? Who chose the child's name?
Does it have special meaning? Who else is called like this? At
which ages do you typically expect a child to wean? To walk? To
speak? To complete toilet training? What activities do you expect a
child of his age to be able to do independently? How do you discipline him? At what age should a child participate in chores? Play
alone? Participate in religious observances? Stay home alone?
How should a child of his age express respect? What kind of eye
contact and physical contact should a child of his age have with
adults? How should a child of his age behave around girls? How
should he dress around them? What languages are spoken at home?
At school? In what ways are religion, spirituality, and community
important in family life? How would you expect this child to participate in these activities?*

Early Development and Home Background

If the CFI helps a practitioner understand the cultural background of a young person and his caregivers, the Early Development and Home Background (EDHB) form helps a
practitioner assess the risks of adverse childhood experiences
(Figures 10–3 and 10–4). Adverse childhood experiences increase the risk of a person experiencing delays in language
acquisition (Vernon-Feagans et al. 2012), having fragmenta-
tion of identity (Scott et al. 2014), underperforming in educational settings (Romano et al. 2015), and developing
substance use disorders (Buu et al. 2009) and mental illnesses
(Dvir et al. 2014).

Adverse childhood experiences are common and are associated with profound health outcomes. Approximately
12.5% of the U.S. general public reports experiencing 4 or
more of the following 10 adverse childhood experiences:
emotional, physical, or sexual abuse; emotional neglect;
physical neglect; physically aggressive mother; household
substance abuse; household mental illness; parental separation or divorce; and incarceration of a household member.
Researchers have linked exposure to such adversities to
long-term changes in self-care and health behaviors. Persons
exposed to 4 or more different types of adverse childhood experiences are more than twice as likely as those without such

Child's Name: _____ Age: ____ Sex: ☐ Male ☐ Female Date: ____

Instructions to Parent or Guardian: Questions P1–P19 ask about the early development and early and current home experiences of your child. Some questions require that you think as far back as to the birth of your child. Your response to these questions will help your child's clinician better understand and care for your child. Answer each question to the best of your knowledge or memory.

What is your relationship with the child receiving care? _____

Please choose one response (✓ or x) for each question.

Early Development	No	Yes	Can't Remember	Don't Know
P1. Was he/she born before he/she was due (premature)?	☐	☐	☐	☐
P2. Were the doctors worried about his/her medical condition immediately after he/she was born?	☐	☐	☐	☐
P3. Did he/she have to spend any time in a neonatal intensive care unit (NICU)?	☐	☐	☐	☐
P4. Could he/she walk on his/her own by the age of 18 months?	☐	☐	☐	☐
P5. Has he/she ever had a seizure?	☐	☐	☐	☐
P6. Did he/she ever lose consciousness for more than a few minutes after an accident?	☐	☐	☐	☐

FIGURE 10–3. Early Development and Home Background (EDHB) form—Parent/Guardian.

Early Communication		No	Yes	Can't Remember	Don't Know
P7.	By the time he/she was age 2, could he/she put several words together when speaking?	❑	❑	❑	❑
P8.	Could people who didn't know him/her understand his/her speech by the time he/she reached age 4?	❑	❑	❑	❑
P9.	Have you ever been concerned about his/her hearing or eyesight?	❑	❑	❑	❑
P10.	By the time he/she was age 4, was he/she interested in playing with or being with other children?	❑	❑	❑	❑

FIGURE 10–3. Early Development and Home Background (EDHB) form—Parent/Guardian. *(continued)*

Home Environment	No	Yes	Can't Remember	Don't Know
P11. Was there ever a time when he/she could not live at home and someone else had to look after him/her?	☐	☐		☐
P12. Has he/she ever been admitted to the hospital for a serious illness?	☐	☐	☐	☐
P13. Does anyone at home suffer from a serious health problem?	☐	☐		☐
P14. Does anyone at home have a problem with depression?	☐	☐		☐
P15. Does anyone at home regularly see a counselor, therapist, or other mental health professional?	☐	☐		☐
P16. Does anyone at home have a problem with alcohol, drugs, or other substances?	☐	☐		☐
P17. Would you say that the atmosphere at home is usually pretty calm?	☐	☐		☐

	Less Than Once a Month	Between Once a Week and Once a Month	More Than Once a Week	Most Days
P18. How often are there fights or arguments between people at home?	☐	☐	☐	☐
P19. How often does your child get criticized to his/her face by other family members when he/she is at home?	☐	☐	☐	☐

FIGURE 10–3. Early Development and Home Background (EDHB) form—Parent/Guardian. *(continued)*

(This form is to be completed if this is your **FIRST** encounter with the child receiving care)

Child's Name: _____ Age: _____ Sex: ☐ Male ☐ Female Date: _____

GENERAL INSTRUCTIONS: The Early Development and Home Background (EDHB) form is used for the assessment of the early development and past and current home background experiences of the child receiving care. The form consists of two versions: 1) 19 P-items, to be completed by the child's parent or guardian, and 2) 8 C-items (herein), to be completed by the clinician. First, the P-items should be completed by the child's parent or guardian. This can be done independently, prior to meeting with the clinician, or be administered to the parent or guardian by the clinician during the clinical interview with the parent's or guardian's response to each question recorded verbatim. Next, the clinician is asked to complete the C-items after a thorough review of the parent's or guardian's responses, ask follow-up questions if necessary, and review any additional clinical information that is available.

Please review the responses provided by the child's parent or guardian for items P1–P10 and then, based on all the information available (i.e., parent/guardian's responses, other information available, and information obtained from the clinical interview), complete questions C1–C4 below

Early CNS Problems

C1.	Is there a history suggestive of early neurological damage?	☐ No	☐ Yes	☐ *Unsure*
If yes, specify:				
C2.	Does history suggest delayed language development?	☐ No	☐ Yes	☐ *Unsure*
C3.	Does history suggest possible persistent problems with vision or hearing?	☐ No	☐ Yes	☐ *Unsure*
C4.	Does history suggest early difficulties in social relationships?	☐ No	☐ Yes	☐ *Unsure*
If yes to any, elaborate:				

FIGURE 10–4. Early Development and Home Background (EDHB) form—Clinician.

Please review the responses provided by the child's parent or guardian for items P11–P16 and then, based on all the information available (i.e., parent/guardian's responses, other information available, and information obtained from the clinical interview), complete questions C5a–d below.

Early Disturbances of Home Environment: Early Abuse or Neglect

C5.	Does history suggest early…			
a.	physical abuse?	❏ No	❏ Yes	❏ *Unsure*
b.	sexual abuse?	❏ No	❏ Yes	❏ *Unsure*
c.	neglect?	❏ No	❏ Yes	❏ *Unsure*
d.	damaging nurturance (e.g. frequent change of caregiver)?	❏ No	❏ Yes	❏ *Unsure*

If yes to any, elaborate:

FIGURE 10–4. Early Development and Home Background (EDHB) form—Clinician. (*continued*)

Please review the response provided by the child's parent or guardian for items P13–P19 and then, based on all the information available (i.e., parent/guardian's responses, other information available, and information obtained from the clinical interview), complete questions C6–C8 below.

Home Environment

		Normal	Somewhat High	High	Very High	Unsure
C6.	Levels of expressed emotion (arguments, expressions of dislike among family members, or criticism of child's behavior, feelings, or individual characteristics) at home are probably ...	☐ Normal	☐ Somewhat High	☐ High	☐ Very High	☐ Unsure
C7.	Is parent/caregiver currently depressed?	☐ No	☐ Somewhat but Mild	☐ Significant	☐ Severe	☐ Unsure

IF ANY ANSWER OTHER THAN "NO" TO QUESTION 7:

C8.	If depressed, is parent/caregiver receiving treatment?	☐ No	☐ Yes	☐ Unsure

FIGURE 10–4. Early Development and Home Background (EDHB) form—Clinician. *(continued)*

experiences to have had a stroke, twice as likely to have ischemic heart disease, 4 times as likely to use illicit substances, 7 times as likely to develop alcoholism, and 12 times as likely to attempt suicide. Improving a child's early household experiences therefore is believed to improve his long-term physical health.

Practitioners often neglect to assess for a history of adverse childhood experiences. After all, keeping up with the demands of the current encounter with a child or an adolescent is challenging enough without also keeping up with events from the past. We encourage you to develop strategies for assessing adverse experiences, both because of the possibility that adverse experiences may be ongoing and because of the certainty that the sequelae of any adverse experiences are still being worked out by the patient. Either way, you will be able to intervene only if you first identify the adverse experiences. The EDHB is one way to do so.

The EDHB is a pair of single-page questionnaires that a practitioner administers sequentially. A caregiver should complete the 19-question version, assessing development, communication, and the home environment, before (or while) the practitioner meets with the patient. An eight-question version, assessing early central nervous system problems, early disturbances in a child's life, and the current home environment, should be completed in an interview of the caregiver.

The EDHB can be reproduced, without additional permission, for a practitioner's clinical use.

Personality Inventory for DSM-5—Brief Form—Child Age 11–17

During the decade of work preceding the publication of DSM-5, most observers anticipated that the personality disorders would be substantially revised. After all, the categorical model of personality disorders has several known problems: many persons with mental illness meet the criteria for several different personality disorders, practitioners often use personality diagnoses pejoratively, the "clustering" of personality disorders has little biological basis, and the categorical model does not allow for the identification of character traits that affect function without constituting a full disorder.

To address these concerns, the authors of DSM-5 created a dimensional model of personality disorders. Unlike a categorical model, in which a practitioner diagnoses a disorder on the basis of the presence of symptoms that negatively affect functioning, in the dimensional model, a practitioner first assesses whether a person has significant deficits in self-functioning and interpersonal functioning before identifying the character traits associated with the functional deficits.

The organizing principle of the dimensional model of personality disorders is called the "five factors." In the literature, *five-factor model* usually refers to the adaptive personality traits of neuroticism, extroversion, agreeableness, conscientiousness, and openness to experience (Digman 1990). Because the DSM-5 Work Group built these diagnostic criteria from a deficit-based rather than a strength-based model, they organized personality disorders around five companion maladaptive traits: negative affect, detachment, antagonism, disinhibition, and psychoticism. The authors found compelling evidence for these five maladaptive traits as stable and predictive of problems in self-functioning and interpersonal functioning. In addition, they identified "facets" for each of these five maladaptive traits. In total, they enumerated 25 facets organized into 5 domains for each of the maladaptive traits listed earlier. The model was accompanied by a Level of Personality Functioning Scale and Personality Trait Rating Form, with which a practitioner could rate the severity of functional impairment and specify a person's maladaptive traits.

If that sounds complicated to you, you are not alone. In the initial version of DSM-5, the dimensional model of personality disorders was tabled in favor of the customary categorical models, with 10 personality disorders organized into Clusters A, B, and C. However, the dimensional model was included in Section III of DSM-5, along with other "Emerging Measures and Models." Many observers believe that a simplified version of the dimensional model for personality disorders will ultimately displace the categorical model.

In the meantime, the authors of DSM-5 have encouraged practitioners to use various tools generated during the creation of the dimensional model for personality disorders. Intriguingly, one of those models is of particular interest to practitioners who care for children and adolescents. Unlike the categorical model, which is designed only for adults, the dimensional model allows for a practitioner to assess for self-functioning and interpersonal functioning and specific mal-adaptive traits in a young person between ages 11 and 17.

The Personality Inventory for DSM-5 is available in versions for both adults and children. The full version for children includes 220 questions to be self-completed by the child or adolescent being evaluated. This version is best used in mental health specialty practices and is available online at www.psychiatry.org/practice/dsm/dsm5/online-assessment-measures.

There is also a brief self-administered version, with only 25 questions, that could be used in general settings by interested practitioners. This version can be used to assess a young person's personality traits over time. The Personality Inventory for DSM-5—Brief Form (Figure 10–5) assesses the five personality trait domains described earlier—negative affect, detachment, antagonism, disinhibition, and psychoticism—along with their associated facets.

To score the Personality Inventory for DSM-5—Brief Form, you sum up a patient's responses. Possible scores range from 0 to 75, with higher scores indicating greater overall personality dysfunction. Further scoring information is available online.

Name: _____   Age: _____   Sex: ☐ Male ☐ Female   Date: _____

Instructions: This is a list of things different people might say about themselves. We are interested in how you would describe yourself. There are no right or wrong answers. So you can describe yourself as honestly as possible, we will keep your responses confidential. We'd like you to take your time and read each statement carefully, selecting the response that best describes you.

		Very False or Often False	Sometimes or Somewhat False	Sometimes or Somewhat True	Very True or Often True	Clinician Use Item score
1	People would describe me as reckless.	0	1	2	3	
2	I feel like I act totally on impulse.	0	1	2	3	
3	Even though I know better, I can't stop making rash decisions.	0	1	2	3	
4	I often feel like nothing I do really matters.	0	1	2	3	
5	Others see me as irresponsible.	0	1	2	3	
6	I'm not good at planning ahead.	0	1	2	3	
7	My thoughts often don't make sense to others.	0	1	2	3	
8	I worry about almost everything.	0	1	2	3	
9	I get emotional easily, often for very little reason.	0	1	2	3	
10	I fear being alone in life more than anything else.	0	1	2	3	

FIGURE 10–5. The Personality Inventory for DSM-5—Brief Form (PID-5-BF)—Child Age 11–17.

		Very False or Often False	Sometimes or Somewhat False	Sometimes or Somewhat True	Very True or Often True	Item score
11	I get stuck on one way of doing things, even when it's clear it won't work.	0	1	2	3	
12	I have seen things that weren't really there.	0	1	2	3	
13	I steer clear of romantic relationships.	0	1	2	3	
14	I'm not interested in making friends.	0	1	2	3	
15	I get irritated easily by all sorts of things.	0	1	2	3	
16	I don't like to get too close to people.	0	1	2	3	
17	It's no big deal if I hurt other peoples' feelings.	0	1	2	3	
18	I rarely get enthusiastic about anything.	0	1	2	3	
19	I crave attention.	0	1	2	3	
20	I often have to deal with people who are less important than me.	0	1	2	3	

FIGURE 10–5. The Personality Inventory for DSM-5—Brief Form (PID-5-BF)—Child Age 11–17. (continued)

		Very False or Often False	Sometimes or Somewhat False	Sometimes or Somewhat True	Very True or Often True	Item score
21	I often have thoughts that make sense to me but that other people say are strange.	0	1	2	3	
22	I use people to get what I want.	0	1	2	3	
23	I often "zone out" and then suddenly come to and realize that a lot of time has passed.	0	1	2	3	
24	Things around me often feel unreal, or more real than usual.	0	1	2	3	
25	It is easy for me to take advantage of others.	0	1	2	3	
					Total/Partial Raw Score:	
					Prorated Total Score: (if 1–6 items left unanswered)	
					Average Total Score:	

FIGURE 10–5. The Personality Inventory for DSM-5—Brief Form (PID-5-BF)—Child Age 11–17. *(continued)*

Chapter 11

Rating Scales and Alternative Diagnostic Systems

There are many ways to describe and measure mental distress. In DSM-5 (American Psychiatric Association 2013), the primary way to do so is by identifying a group of symptoms that impair a person's psychosocial function. These symptoms follow each other in predictable ways, and we call these collections of functionally impairing systems *mental disorders*. DSM-5 mental disorders are diagnostic labels rather than discrete biological phenomena. Within a particular diagnosis, there are very different experiences of symptoms and functional impairment. One adolescent with major depressive disorder may need coping strategies, whereas another may need hospitalization. To account for these differences, we can measure a young person's areas of mental distress with rating scales. Sometimes, we also use alternative diagnostic systems as a way to describe the distress differently.

Because we cannot yet diagnose and monitor mental illness through means such as physical diagnosis, functional imaging, genetic testing, or blood serum tests, rating scales are important aids to clinical care. Individual item responses on a rating scale can be used to guide a clinical conversation: "You indicated that you sometimes have thoughts that you would be better off dead…can you tell me more about that?" Numerical scores on rating scales identify symptoms, guide diagnostic assessments, establish the severity of a disorder, and track the progress of a young person's care. Collecting rating scale results over time also will enable measurement-based care, which refers to adjusting a patient's treatment plan until a measurable symptom target is reached.

We follow a few principles when considering how to use rating scales:

- Select scales that are research validated for age, condition, and (ideally) culture.
- Use broad-based screening scales to detect the likelihood of any disorder being present.
- Use a more specific rating scale to investigate a particular problem.
- Select brief rating scales to enhance patient cooperation and ease of implementation.
- Reserve longer rating scales for specialty settings.
- Note that rating scales cannot make diagnoses—they are aids, not replacements, for clinician assessments.
- Remember that rating scale results depend on the reliability of the reporter and her interpretation.

Many scales are copyrighted by their authors and thus are not freely available. Table 11–1 contains a list of freely available rating scales in common use that have been research validated for use with young people. In this context, validity means that each scale has a research-supported scoring system that balances the need for good sensitivity (the test detects most patients who have a disorder) and good specificity (the test is positive only when a disorder is present).

DSM-5 provides severity rating scales for many disorders. Most of these scales are specific to a particular disorder, and some include a narrative description to indicate that a particular disorder is mild, moderate, or severe. For some diagnoses, such as alcohol use disorder, severity depends on the number of criteria endorsed by a patient. In other instances, severity is measured by the degree to which a patient requires support, as in autism spectrum disorder. When appropriate, the severity ratings refer to specific measurements external to your mental status examination. For example, one aspect of assessing the severity of intellectual disability entails assessing a patient's IQ.

The authors of DSM-5 have posted several disorder-specific severity measures (Table 11–2) at www.psychiatry.org/practice/dsm/dsm5/online-assessment-measures. These measures can be used (and reproduced) for clinical and research evaluation without further permission. A practitioner who frequently cares for children and adolescents with these specific conditions should consider using them in her practice.

TABLE 11–1. Selected brief rating scales that are validated and free to use with children and adolescents

Category	Scale	Number of items	Validated ages for use (years)
Overall psychosocial difficulties	Pediatric Symptom Checklist (PSC, PSC-17)	Parent: 35 or 17 Youth: 35	4–17 (parent version) 11–17 (youth version)
	Strengths and Difficulties Questionnaire (SDQ)	Parent: 25	4–16
Global functioning	Columbia Impairment Scale	Parent: 13 Youth: 13	9–17
	Brief Impairment Scale	Parent: 21	4–17
Behavior and emotional development	Early Childhood Screening Assessment (ECSA)	Parent: 40	1.5–5
Anxiety	Screen for Child Anxiety Related Emotional Disorders (SCARED)	Parent and youth: 41	9–17
	Spence Children's Anxiety Scale (SCAS)	Parent: 39 Youth: 45	6–17
	Spence Preschool Anxiety Scale	Parent: 39	3–5

TABLE 11–1. Selected brief rating scales that are validated and free to use with children and adolescents *(continued)*

Category	Scale	Number of items	Validated ages for use (years)
Depression	Short Mood and Feelings Questionnaire (SMFQ)	Parent: 13 Youth: 13	8–17
	Patient Health Questionnaire-9 (PHQ-9)	Youth: 9	13–17
	Center for Epidemiologic Studies Depression Scale for Children (CES-DC)	Youth: 20	13–17
Attention-deficit disorder, attention-deficit/hyperactivity disorder	Vanderbilt ADHD Diagnostic Parent Rating Scale/Vanderbilt ADHD Diagnostic Teacher Rating Scale	Parent: 55 Teacher: 43	6–12
	SNAP-IV-C Rating Scale	Parent/teacher: 90	6–17
	ADHD Rating Scale-IV	Parent/teacher: 18	6–17
Posttraumatic stress disorder	Children's Revised Impact of Events Scale-8 (CRIES-8)	Youth: 8	8–17
Substance use	CRAFFT (Car, Relax, Alone, Forget, Friends, Trouble)	Youth: 6	13–17

TABLE 11–1. Selected brief rating scales that are validated and free to use with children and adolescents (*continued*)

Category	Scale	Number of items	Validated ages for use (years)
Autism spectrum disorder	Modified Checklist for Autism in Toddlers (M-CHAT)	Parent: 23	16–30 months
	Childhood Autism Spectrum Test (CAST)	Parent: 39	4–11
	Autism-Spectrum Quotient (AQ)	Parent: 50	12–15
Maternal depression	Edinburgh Postnatal Depression Scale (EPDS)	Parent: 10	Peripartum women

TABLE 11–2. DSM-5 disorder-specific severity measures for children and adolescents, ages 11–17 years

Rater	Scale	Number of items	Source measure
Self	Severity Measure for Depression	9	Adapted from PHQ-9 modified for adolescents (PHQ-A)
Self	Severity Measure for Separation Anxiety Disorder	10	Each anxiety severity scale contains the same 10 items, with a few phrasing adaptations to match the DSM-5 criteria for each disorder
Self	Severity Measure for Specific Phobia	10	
Self	Severity Measure for Social Anxiety Disorder (Social Phobia)	10	
Self	Severity Measure for Panic Disorder	10	
Self	Severity Measure for Agoraphobia	10	
Self	Severity Measure for Generalized Anxiety Disorder	10	
Self	Severity of Posttraumatic Stress Symptoms	9	National Stressful Events Survey PTSD Short Scale (NSESS)
Self	Severity of Acute Stress Symptoms	7	National Stressful Events Survey Acute Stress Disorder Short Scale (NSESS)

TABLE 11–2. DSM-5 disorder-specific severity measures for children and adolescents, ages 11–17 years *(continued)*

Rater	Scale	Number of items	Source measure
Self	Severity of Dissociative Symptoms	8	Brief Dissociative Experiences Scale (DES-B)
Practitioner	Clinician-Rated Severity of Autism Spectrum and Social Communication Disorders	2	Uses DSM-5 autism severity descriptions
Practitioner	Clinician-Rated Dimensions of Psychosis Symptom Severity	8	Not adapted: appears in Section III of DSM-5
Practitioner	Clinician-Rated Severity of Somatic Symptom Disorder	3	Derived from DSM-5 disorder diagnostic criteria
Practitioner	Clinician-Rated Severity of Oppositional Defiant Disorder	1	Uses DSM-5 oppositional defiant disorder severity description
Practitioner	Clinician-Rated Severity of Conduct Disorder	1	Uses DSM-5 conduct disorder severity description
Practitioner	Clinician-Rated Severity of Nonsuicidal Self-Injury	1	Derived from DSM-5 diagnostic threshold for proposed nonsuicidal self-injury disorder

Alternative Diagnostic Systems

Although DSM-5 has been widely adopted, it is not the only way practitioners can describe and account for mental distress and mental illness. In different cultural and clinical situations, the following diagnostic systems are in use.

International Classification of Diseases

The World Health Organization maintains its own diagnostic system, the International Classification of Diseases, commonly known by its abbreviation, ICD. The current, tenth edition (ICD-10; World Health Organization 1992) includes mental disorders among a catalog of all medical diseases. The eleventh edition is under development and is due for release in 2017. Although most clinicians outside the United States use ICD-10 to diagnose mental disorders, ICD-10 is less psychiatrically detailed than DSM-5 and was designed primarily to help epidemiologists track the incidence and prevalence of disease. Despite having different designs, DSM-5 and ICD-10 assign the same codes to psychiatric diagnoses and thus are in shared use by insurers. For example, if a practitioner diagnoses DSM-5 autism spectrum disorder in a child, the diagnosis shares a diagnostic code with ICD-10 childhood autism disorder. You can find more information about ICD-10 and a list of diagnostic codes at www.who.int/classifications/icd/en, and the fifth chapter of ICD-10, "Mental and Behavioral Disorders," includes most of the relevant diagnoses.

Research Domain Criteria

In 2010, the National Institute of Mental Health announced its intention to produce its own diagnostic system, the Research Domain Criteria (RDoC), which will attempt to unite symptoms with their underlying causes (Insel et al. 2010). At present, RDoC serves as an experimental framework for researching the biological origin of psychiatric illness, so it cannot yet replace any current clinical diagnostic system. The ultimate goal of this project is to map behavioral patterns onto particular neural circuits, cells, genes, or molecules for which new research and new treatments could be developed. In this way, a specific behavioral pattern such as impulsivity, which is a trait that may occur in many different current

DSM-5 diagnoses, might be found through the RDoC to have a relatively unified underlying biological cause. You can follow the progress of the development of the RDoC at www.nimh.nih.gov/research-priorities/rdoc/index.shtml.

Culture-Specific Diagnostic Systems

Several culture-specific psychiatric diagnostic systems are used in particular communities, including Latin America (Berganza et al. 2002), Cuba (Otero-Ojeda 2002), China (Chen 2002), and Japan (Nakane and Nakane 2002). There is also a French diagnostic system specifically designed for use with children and adolescents (Mises et al. 2002).

Diagnostic Systems for Infants and Toddlers

Several diagnostic systems exist for assessing psychopathology in very young children (Egger and Emde 2011). The most widely used, the *Diagnostic Classification of Mental Health and Developmental Disorders of Infancy and Early Childhood* (DC:0–3), was published in 1994 for the evaluation of children ages 0–3 years (Zero to Three 1994). A revised edition, *Diagnostic Classification of Mental Health and Developmental Disorders of Infancy and Early Childhood, Revised* (DC:0–3R), is also available (Zero to Three 2005). It uses a five-axis system as in DSM-IV (American Psychiatric Association 1994) but is shaped around describing infant relationships and problematic behavior patterns. The Research Diagnostic Criteria–Preschool Age (RDC-PA) was designed for the evaluation of children ages 0–5 years participating in behavioral health research (Task Force on Research Diagnostic Criteria: Infancy Preschool 2003).

ICD-10 Z Codes

DSM-5 recommends the use of ICD-10 Z codes as a way to account for the psychosocial factors that are currently affecting a young person's mental health and treatment. ICD-10 Z codes are discussed further in Chapter 13, "Mental Health Treatment Planning," but we are including a truncated list in Table 11–3.

TABLE 11–3. ICD-10 codes commonly used in child and adolescent mental health

ICD-10 code	Description
Z00.4	General psychiatric examination, not elsewhere classified Exclusion: examination requested for medicolegal reasons (Z04.6)
Z04.6	General psychiatric examination, requested by authority
Z30.0	General counseling and advice on contraception
Z33	Pregnant state, incidental
Z50.2	Alcohol rehabilitation
Z50.3	Drug rehabilitation
Z50.4	Psychotherapy, not elsewhere classified
Z51.5	Palliative care
Z55.0	Illiteracy and low-level literacy
Z55.3	Underachievement in school
Z55.4	Educational maladjustment and discord with teachers and classmates
Z55.9	Academic or educational problem
Z59.0	Homelessness
Z59.1	Inadequate housing
Z59.2	Discord with neighbor, lodger, or landlord
Z59.3	Problem related to living in a residential institution
Z59.4	Lack of adequate food or safe drinking water
Z59.5	Extreme poverty
Z59.6	Low income
Z59.7	Insufficient social insurance or welfare support
Z79.9	Unspecified housing or economic problem
Z60.0	Phase of life problem
Z60.3	Acculturation difficulty
Z60.4	Social exclusion or rejection
Z60.5	Target of (perceived) adverse discrimination or persecution

TABLE 11–3. ICD-10 codes commonly used in child and adolescent mental health *(continued)*

ICD-10 code	Description
Z60.9	Unspecified problem related to social environment
Z61.0	Loss of love relationship in childhood
Z61.1	Removal from home in childhood
Z61.2	Altered pattern of family relationships in childhood
Z61.3	Events resulting in loss of self-esteem in childhood
Z61.4	Problems related to alleged sexual abuse of child by person within primary support group
Z61.5	Problems related to alleged sexual abuse of child by person outside primary support group
Z61.6	Problems related to alleged physical abuse of child
Z61.7	Personal frightening experience in childhood
Z62.0	Inadequate parental supervision and control
Z62.1	Parental overprotection
Z62.2	Institutional upbringing
Z62.4	Emotional neglect of child
Z62.820	Parent-child relational problem
Z62.891	Sibling relational problem
Z62.29	Upbringing away from parents
Z62.810	Personal history (past history) of physical abuse in childhood
Z62.810	Personal history (past history) of sexual abuse in childhood
Z62.811	Personal history (past history) of psychological abuse in childhood
Z62.812	Personal history (past history) of neglect in childhood
Z62.898	Child affected by parental relationship distress

TABLE 11–3. ICD-10 codes commonly used in child and adolescent mental health *(continued)*

ICD-10 code	Description
Z63.1	Problems in relationship with parents and in-laws
Z63.2	Inadequate family support
Z63.4	Uncomplicated bereavement
Z63.5	Disruption of family by separation or divorce
Z63.6	Dependent relative needing care at home
Z63.8	High expressed emotion level within family
Z64.0	Problems related to unwanted pregnancy
Z64.1	Problems related to multiparity
Z64.2	Seeking and acceptin3g physical, nutritional and chemical interventions known to be hazardous and harmful Exclusion: substance dependence
Z64.3	Seeking and accepting behavioural and psychological interventions known to be hazardous and harmful
Z64.4	Discord with social service provider, including probation officer, case manager, or social services worker
Z65.0	Conviction in civil and criminal proceedings without imprisonment
Z65.1	Imprisonment or other incarceration
Z65.2	Problems related to release from prison
Z65.3	Problems related to other legal circumstances
Z65.4	Victim of crime or terrorism
Z65.5	Exposure to disaster, war, or other hostilities
Z65.8	Other problem related to psychosocial circumstances
Z65.8	Religious or spiritual problem
Z65.9	Unspecified problem related to unspecified psychosocial circumstances
Z69.010	Encounter for mental health services for victim of child abuse or neglect by parent

TABLE 11–3. ICD-10 codes commonly used in child and adolescent mental health *(continued)*

ICD-10 code	Description
Z69.020	Encounter for mental health services for victim of nonparental child abuse or neglect
Z70.3	Counselling related to combined concerns regarding sexual attitude, behaviour and orientation
Z71.1	Person with feared complaint in whom no diagnosis is made
Z71.4	Alcohol abuse counselling and surveillance Exclusion: alcohol rehabilitation procedures
Z71.5	Drug abuse counselling and surveillance Exclusion: drug rehabilitation procedures
Z71.6	Tobacco abuse counseling Exclusion: tobacco rehabilitation procedures
Z72.0	Tobacco use disorder, mild
Z72.1	Alcohol use Exclusion: alcohol dependence
Z72.2	Drug use Exclusion: abuse of non-dependence-producing substances, drug dependence
Z72.3	Lack of physical exercise
Z72.4	Inappropriate diet and eating habits Exclusion: eating disorder or lack of food
Z72.5	High-risk sexual behaviour
Z72.810	Child or adolescent antisocial behavior
Z73.6	Limitation of activities due to disability Exclusion: care-provider dependency
Z74.0	Reduced mobility
Z74.1	Need for assistance with personal care
Z74.3	Need for continuous supervision
Z75.1	Person awaiting admission to adequate facility elsewhere
Z75.3	Unavailability or inaccessibility of health care facilities

TABLE 11–3. ICD-10 codes commonly used in child and adolescent mental health *(continued)*

ICD-10 code	Description
Z75.4	Unavailability or inaccessibility of other helping agencies
Z76.5	Malingering
Z91.1	Personal history of noncompliance with medical treatment and regimen
Z71.2	Nonadherence to medical treatment
Z91.2	Personal history of poor personal hygiene
Z91.3	Personal history of unhealthy sleep-wake schedule
Z71.49	Other personal history of psychological trauma
Z91.5	Personal history of self-harm
Z91.6	Personal history of other physical trauma
Z71.83	Wandering associated with a mental disorder
T74.02XA T74.02XD	Child neglect, confirmed , Initial encounter , Subsequent encounter
T76.02XA T76.02XD	Child neglect, suspected , Initial encounter , Subsequent encounter
T74.32XA T74.32XD	Child psychological abuse, confirmed , Initial encounter , Subsequent encounter
T76.32XA T76.32XD	Child psychological abuse, suspected , Initial encounter , Subsequent encounter
T74.22XA T74.22XD	Child sexual abuse, confirmed , Initial encounter , Subsequent encounter
T76.22XA T76.22XD	Child sexual abuse, suspected , Initial encounter , Subsequent encounter

Chapter 12

Developmental Milestones

Observations of child maturation by developmental theorists are foundational for pediatrics, child psychiatry, and child psychology. The work of many different theorists over the years (e.g., Beloglovsky and Daly 2015; McCartney and Philips 2006; Mooney 2013) has resulted in a diverse set of child developmental theories that are intended to help us understand what happens during child development. Surveying the entirety of this literature is beyond the scope of this text. Instead, we discuss specific observable milestones within child development and their recognized patterns of appearance.

Milestones are recognizable skills or abilities that have an expected range and order of appearance, such as a child taking his first step around the time of his first birthday. Identifying any significant variations from expected patterns, such as a child taking that first step near his second birthday, is a key task for any practitioner. Knowing when a significant variation in development has occurred improves diagnostic accuracy because DSM-5 (American Psychiatric Association 2013) specifically requires consideration of developmental stages. The most important consideration is that the sooner a significant developmental impairment is identified and addressed, the better the long-term outcomes could be for your patients.

Identifying milestones is a particularly important skill set for practitioners working with children younger than 5 years, but we all need to be familiar with milestones because nonsevere developmental impairments frequently go unrecognized until children are much older. Five different milestone skill areas should be evaluated: gross/fine motor, visual motor problem solving, speech and language, social/emotional, and adaptive skills (Gerber et al. 2011).

Gross motor skills are the most obvious to recognize because they involve crawling, walking, running, and throwing. Early motor skills are about performing basic body control tasks, starting with first maintaining a head position, then moving the trunk, followed by moving the whole body in ever more skillful ways. Besides significant delays in gross motor skills, any physical findings of abnormal reflexes, asymmetric muscle tone, or being too loose or too tight in overall muscle tone are other gross motor abnormalities that should be noted.

Visual motor problem solving describes a child's physical interactions with the world. Infants begin by visually tracking and following people or objects, then reaching for and manipulating objects, and later acquire the ability to draw and to write. These fine motor skills (using one's hands and fingers) rely on visual input and generally progress at a slower pace than gross motor skills. If the development of these milestones is delayed, it may be because of impairments in sensory, cognitive, or motor abilities.

Speech and language skills are essential for social interactions and academic success. To be able to communicate, a person first has to be able to receive input (process what is seen and heard), pragmatically understand the meaning of that input, then generate an expression of his thoughts (translate thoughts into words, then express fluently). Delays in expressive language milestones may be more apparent than receptive language delays, which may be more subtle but when present may worsen an expressive language impairment.

Social/emotional skills are the core elements of psychiatric functioning. Infants are essentially born with three emotions (anger, joy, and fear), and the circumstances to elicit those feelings become increasingly complex as they grow up. Social skill development is interactive and thus reliant on the presence of a responsive caregiver. A child's temperamental traits, such as having a high- or low-intensity disposition, influence how he responds to routine activities, which influences how his caregivers respond. Developing shared joint attention with another person by approximately age 1 year is a key social milestone. Normal social and emotional development relies on many other skills but is most closely linked with speech and language skills.

Adaptive skills initially involve learning to feed oneself, dress oneself, and use the bathroom. For older children, adaptive skills involve self-direction, self-protection, and the ability to function independently in a school setting. Adaptive skills use both motor and cognitive abilities and thus are not a truly independent category of development. When you evaluate for the presence of an intellectual disability, adaptive milestones need to be investigated because the intellectual disability diagnosis should not be made without demonstrable impairments in adaptive functioning. Standardized intelligence testing is no longer considered the sole basis for diagnosing intellectual disability.

A child may acquire all of his skills in the usual sequence but at a slower rate (a delay), may acquire his skills at differential rates in different areas (a dissociation), or may achieve milestones out of the usual order of acquisition (a deviation). Growth and development will follow recognizable patterns, but it is not an exact script. For instance, a perfectly healthy child might never crawl, instead scooting or rolling to move around before taking his first steps. The task of a pediatric health care practitioner is to always consider what would constitute normal-range development (Table 12–1). Then he can, variously, alert caregivers if a child is not keeping pace with development and thus needs developmental assistance services, reassure worried caregivers when a child is keeping pace with the normal range of development, or simply better understand how a child engages his environment.

Determining when a child's delayed milestone acquisition would indicate the need for further evaluations or an intervention can be a challenging decision when developmental delays are subtle. To guide your decision, Table 12–2 contains a list of specific cognitive, motor, and social/emotional traits at different ages that suggest a need to refer for specialized developmental assessments.

TABLE 12–1. Selected normal-range developmental milestones

Age	Gross motor	Visual motor	Speech and language	Social/emotional	Adaptive skills
2 months	Has good head control; lifts chest up in prone	Tracks with eyes; holds own hands	Is alert to voice; makes vowel-like noises	Shows reciprocal smiling; recognizes parents	Opens mouth at sight of breast or bottle
4 months	Leans on wrists in prone; rolls prone to supine	Has hands usually open; reaches persistently	Orients self to voice; vocalizes in response	Parent's voice stops cry; smiles on own	Briefly holds breast or bottle
6 months	Briefly sits alone; pivots in prone	Rakes item to pick up; transfers hand to hand	Stops briefly for "no"; babbles consonants	Has stranger anxiety; visually identifies parent	Feeds self crackers; stares at new faces
9 months	Pulls to stand; cruises; comes to sit	Has immature pincer; looks for fallen toy	Imitates sounds; enjoys gesture games	Follows a point; experiences separation anxiety	Bites, chews cookie; looks for fallen item
12 months	Stands well; takes independent steps	Has fine pincer grasp; scribbles if shown	Follows one-step request; uses gestures	Points to get object; shows shared interest	Finger feeds items; takes off a hat

TABLE 12–1. Selected normal-range developmental milestones *(continued)*

Age	Gross motor	Visual motor	Speech and language	Social/emotional	Adaptive skills
18 months	Runs well; stands for ball throw	Scribbles on own; makes 3-cube tower	Points to self; uses 10–25 words	Can show shame; does pretend play	Gets onto chair; removes garment
2 years	Throws overhand; kicks ball	Makes 4-cube train; imitates circle and line	Uses two-word sentences; understands me and you	Does parallel play; begins defiance	Opens doorknob; pulls off pants
3 years	Walks up stairs; catches ball	Copies a circle; recognizes a color	Uses three-word sentences; names body parts	Engages in imaginative play; can share on own	Begins independent eating; unbuttons item
4 years	Balances on one foot 4 seconds; can broad jump 1 foot	Writes part of name; copies a square	Follows three-step request; tells stories	Group play; has preferred friend	Toilets self alone; uses fork well
5 years	Walks down stairs; jumps backward	Cuts with scissors; uses a paper clip	Responds to "why?"; likes rhyming words	Apologizes for error; has group of friends	Dresses and bathes independently

Source. Adapted from Gerber et al. 2010a, 2010b, 2011.

TABLE 12–2. Developmental red flags that should trigger specialized assessments

Age	Cognitive	Motor	Social/emotional
4 months	Lack of visual tracking; no laugh or vocalizations	Lack of seated head control; inability to grasp toy	Does not watch/track people; does not have a smile response
6 months	Failure to turn toward sound or voice	Does not roll or move on the floor	Lack of spontaneous smile
9 months	Lack of babbling consonants	Inability to sit	Cannot reciprocate vocalizations or facial expressions
1 year	Cannot respond to own name; cannot use any words	Cannot hold two objects and hit them together; cannot pull to a stand	Cannot reciprocate hand gestures; will not share joint attention ("Look at…")
1.5 years	Cannot point to a named object; cannot use any words	Unable to walk independently	Lack of any speaking/gesture combinations
2 years	Speech much less than 50% understandable	Cannot walk on steps with assistance; cannot kick a ball	Cannot use a meaningful two-word phrase; lack of empathy (looking sad if a child cries)

TABLE 12–2. Developmental red flags that should trigger specialized assessments *(continued)*

Age	Cognitive	Motor	Social/emotional
3 years	Cannot use a three-word sentence; speech only 50% understandable	Cannot jump; cannot throw object overhand	Never imitates adult activities; cannot do parallel play
4 years	Speech less than 75% understandable; cannot identify self or details in pictures	Cannot balance on one foot for 3 seconds; cannot copy a circle	Lack of imaginative play; cannot hypothesize another's thoughts

Source. Adapted from Gerber et al. 2010a, 2010b, 2011; McLaughlin 2011.

Chapter 13

Mental Health Treatment Planning

Treatment plans can be understood as a regulatory requirement, one of the many chores of contemporary health care, or they can be understood as recipes for changing a patient's life. After all, the goal of any medical intervention is to help a person achieve a therapeutic change she cannot make on her own, so a treatment plan simply names what she needs to change, who will help her, and how she will make the change. Any reasonable treatment plan will include a problem list, a list of measurable goals, and a recipe for how to achieve them.

The reality, of course, is that managing a treatment plan is both a recipe and a chore. After all, treatment plans are often mental health care regulatory requirements demanded by governmental agencies and third-party payers. Regulators and payers often require the completion of mental health treatment plans in a proprietary format. We encourage you to identify treatment plans specific to your clinical setting, because only those treatment plans will fulfill the chore aspect of a treatment plan. In this chapter, we discuss three general principles universal to the recipe aspect of treatment plans: problem lists, patient and caregiver goals, and best practices. They are the what, the who, and the how of treatment plans.

Problem Lists

When you evaluate a young person in mental distress, your goal should be to create a therapeutic alliance, but the tangible result of an evaluation is a diagnosis. This diagnosis is the foundation of a treatment plan.

In earlier versions of DSM, diagnoses were described in a multiaxial, or five-axis, system. Practitioners divided a diagnosis into five components: mental disorders, personality disorders, general medical conditions, psychosocial problems, and global functioning. At its best, the multiaxial system encouraged practitioners to understand a person's distress from several different perspectives: a biological account of mental illness, a psychological account of personality, a mechanistic account of physical illness, a subjective list of psychosocial factors, and a standardized assessment of functioning. At its worst, the multiaxial system reinforced divisions between mind and body; allowed personality disorders to be used as pejorative slurs; included inconsistent accounts of psychosocial functioning; and jumbled together categories, lists, and assessments. It turned out to be a messy recipe.

The authors of DSM-5 (American Psychiatric Association 2013) reorganized the multiaxial system into a problem list. For physicians, the problem list is familiar, because it is already in use throughout medicine. Nonphysicians may benefit from a brief introduction to the problem list. Simply put, a problem list is a comprehensive, hierarchical catalog of the problems addressed during a current encounter.

To be helpful, the items on the list should be standardized because standardization enables communication. There are many ways to account for mental distress and mental illness. Individual practitioners may focus on dysfunctional neural circuits, adverse childhood experiences, or maladaptive personality traits. When these practitioners wish to speak with each other, they need a standard list. The standard list we favor is DSM-5 because it is the consensus diagnostic system of contemporary psychiatry, our way for mental health practitioners to work together while we await a diagnostic system with greater validity.

One reminder that we are awaiting a diagnostic system with improved validity is that the diagnoses generated by a DSM-5 interview are called disorders rather than diseases or illnesses. Physicians usually think in terms of diseases, which can be described as pathological abnormalities in the structure and function of body organs and systems. Patients usually present with illnesses, their experience of pathological abnormalities or of being sick. From a distance, diseases and illnesses may seem like the same experience viewed from the different perspectives of patient and physician. However, diseases and illnesses are often divergent experiences, not just different perspectives, as anthropologists have repeatedly documented (Estroff and Henderson 2005).

Disorders are a kind of middle path between disease and illness because the term acknowledges the complex interplay of biological, social, cultural, and psychological factors in mental distress. Broadly speaking, a disorder simply indicates a disturbance in physical or psychological functioning. Use of the disorder label to describe mental distress draws attention to how mental distress impairs a person's functioning, suggests the complex interplay of events that result in mental distress, and implicitly acknowledges the limits of our knowledge about the causes of mental distress (Kendler 2012). The field does not yet know enough to be more precise. The ongoing use of *disorder* in our diagnostic systems is an opportunity for humility and a spur to further study but primarily is a way to communicate together.

In order for DSM-5 to work as a common language, practitioners need to select a specific diagnosis. Standardization does not work without specificity. Imagine a recipe that asks you to add "a serving of fat." Someone following the recipe would be confused. Did the author of the recipe mean a spoonful of bacon drippings, 2 tablespoons of salted butter, or a half-cup of coconut oil? Each is possible, but each results in a different dish. More to the point, it makes the recipe more of a personal inspiration than a communal instruction. Similarly, practitioners should recognize that characterizing a young person as having "an unspecified mental disorder" inadequately communicates the precise nature of a patient's illness to other practitioners.

We encourage practitioners to select the most specific diagnosis for which a patient qualifies. If you believe a child is depressed, determine not only whether the depression constitutes a major depressive episode but also whether it is a single or recurrent episode, with or without psychotic features, and whether it is mild, moderate, or severe. This level of specificity enables communication with other practitioners and informs their treatment. We recognize the different ways to treat depression in a child if it is a mild first episode rather than a severe recurrent episode with psychotic features, but we barely know how to proceed with a child who has a nonspecific disorder. Identifying a specific disorder improves communication with other practitioners, while communicating to your patients (and their caregivers) your diagnostic ability and your understanding of the patient's illness. Diagnosis is, itself, a response to a patient's suffering, because giving a specific name to the seemingly unnamable is itself salutary. (It also improves your ability to communicate with regulators and third-party payers, many of whom reimburse better for more specific diagnoses.)

Still, at times, a specific diagnosis is inappropriate. When you are uncertain of the diagnosis or need additional information, a provisional diagnosis is always preferable to a specific but inaccurate diagnosis. Just remember to eventually arrive at the most specific diagnosis possible. It is discouraging to review medical records in which a young person's diagnosis remains poorly characterized for years.

Even if your diagnoses lack specificity, you can make them comprehensive. They should include all problems that are currently diminishing a young person's ability to function. Thus, the list should include mental disorders, general medical conditions, and psychosocial problems. We, as you know by now, use DSM-5 to describe mental disorders, including the adverse effects from psychiatric treatment that are described in Section II of DSM-5. To describe general medical conditions, we include the medical conditions that are currently affecting a young person's function. You do not need to list well-healed injuries. To describe psychosocial problems that influence a young person's health, we favor using the standardized list of ICD-10 (World Health Organization 1992) Z codes. Several of the most relevant Z codes are found in Chapter 11, "Rating Scales and Alternative Diagnostic Systems," of this book, but the complete list of Z codes, numbered Z00–Z99, is found in the ICD chapter "Factors Influencing Health Status and Contact With Health Services," which can be found online at http://apps.who.int/classifications/icd10/browse/2010/en#/XXI.

Finally, the problems should be ordered hierarchically. Problems that are the focus of your treatment should lead the list. For example, an adolescent may have cystic fibrosis, but if you are treating her for an episode of major depressive disorder following an intentional overdose, then her first two problems are her major depressive disorder and her suicide attempt. If you evaluate her again 2 months later and she has recovered from her depression and has recovered from her overdose, then her depressive episode and suicide attempt would be lower on her problem list. A well-ordered problem list communicates to everyone who reviews your record the focus of your treatment.

Patient and Caregiver Goals

You develop the goals of your treatment in conversation with your patient and her caregivers. Sometimes practitioners ask about goals toward the end of a clinical conversation. We prefer to ask about goals from the beginning and then throughout a conversation. Asking about goals is another way to establish a therapeutic alliance, the mutual commitment you and a patient make to improve her well-being. You and the patient establish the alliance when a patient identifies treatment goals and you ally yourself with her in pursuit of those goals. By doing this early in your encounter, you invariably increase the amount and reliability of information a patient offers. More profoundly, you help motivate a patient's desire to change. We ask, often very directly, "What is your treatment goal?" or with younger children, "If you had three magic wishes, what would you change about your life?" Then, as the encounter progresses, we frequently check about additional goals, saying something like, "I hear that you are concerned; should we address that as a treatment goal?" or for smaller children, "Is that the kind of thing you would use a magic wish on?" By continuing to ask about treatment goals, a practitioner clarifies the focus of treatment and further builds the alliance with a patient.

By the end of a conversation in which you have frequently asked about treatment goals, it is usually straightforward to summarize the most pressing treatment goals. We often do so by saying, "It sounds like we have identified the most important treatment goals, but I want to be certain. Have we identified the right goals?" or with a younger child, "I think I know what you would use your three wishes on, but I want to check with you and be sure." These kinds of conversations ensure that your treatment goals will reflect a patient's desire, which usually increases her interest in pursuing the treatment goals. When possible and appropriate, phrase the treatment goals with the patient's own words.

Part of the challenge of working with children and adolescents with mental distress is bringing patients and caregivers together in pursuit of common goals. With patients, we prefer to identify goals early in an encounter. With caregivers, we like to understand the relationship between a caregiver and a patient before asking about treatment goals. Different caregivers will be invested in a patient in different ways. Is the caregiver a biological parent, stepparent, foster parent, grandparent, older sibling, guardian, probation officer, or teacher? These relationships affect the treatment goals a caregiver identifies and her ability to affect those goals. If, say, an adolescent presents for treatment with her probation officer, the treatment goals will likely include legal requirements, which are quite different from the patient's goals. You need to know how and why a caregiver is involved in a young person's life before soliciting a caregiver's treatment goals.

Once the patient, caregiver, and practitioner agree on treatment goals, it helps to consider the settings in which the goals will be pursued. If the problems you mutually identify occur mostly at home, then the goals should focus on the home. If the problems occur mostly at school, then your goals need to engage the school's teachers and staff. If you are seeing the patient in a primary care clinic, the treatment goal may include learning coping skills, developing new habits, or establishing care with a mental health practitioner. If you are seeing the patient in a hospital, the treatment goals usually address acute concerns, such as decreasing suicidality or improving mood.

Any good treatment goal can be achieved. It does no one a service to set unachievable goals. Unachievable goals are a species of magic thinking, the wish that simply thinking about something will make it happen. We may earnestly desire to play center for an NBA team, but no amount of training will ever help two middle-aged psychiatrists achieve that goal. Similarly, it is foolish to set a goal that is truly impossible for a young person—whether because of age, developmental status, or physical or psychological characteristics—to achieve. It also does no one a service to set unexceptional goals. Unexceptional goals are a kind of everyday cruelty, the setting of the low bar in order to claim an unearned victory. We may not play basketball like NBA centers, but we can (at least for now!) tie our own shoes, so setting a treatment goal of shoelace tying would be insulting. The best goals are just a little bit out of reach of what seems possible; in our hypothetical case, our goal should be to improve our passing and shooting in games of pickup basketball. Pursuing similarly appropriate goals improves the lives of patients, caregivers, and practitioners because these goals expand our imagination for what is possible.

Writing about how setting the right goal can expand our imagination of the possible can seem too aspirational, so we remind you that goals must simultaneously be measurable. A treatment goal cannot be to "be more healthy," "be less ill," or "have better behavior." Parents often say they want their children to be "good," which is a similarly unmeasurable goal. In our own example, a difficult-to-measure goal would be that we each "become a better basketball player," whereas a measurable goal would be to "increase our assist-to-turnover ratio from 1.5 to at least 4.5." The treatment goals you set with patients also should be measurable, so that you know when the patient is, or is not, achieving the goals you have agreed on.

Best Practices

One way to identify achievable and measurable goals is to personalize treatment goals to what is possible to achieve as reported in the medical literature. Several practice guidelines and treatment plans are available (e.g., Nurcombe 2014). In our work with young people, we prefer the practice parameters created and maintained by the American Academy of Child and Adolescent Psychiatry (AACAP). The parameters cover most of the major categories of mental illness that children and adolescents experience. The parameters were written by experts in the field and include information about etiology, diagnosis, treatment, and prognosis. All include specific recommendations that can be widely adopted. The practice parameters can be found online at www.jaacap.com/content/pracparam.

As of this writing, 52 practice parameters are included in the AACAP library. We could never hope to summarize all 52 here. Even if we could, they are dynamic documents, and some of them will likely have been updated by the time you read this text. Instead, we dispersed some of the knowledge in the current practice parameters throughout this book, especially in the next three chapters. The American Psychiatric Association also has developed a set of clinical practice guidelines, but these are targeted to treatment in adult patients. Those guidelines of care may be found at http://psychiatryonline.org/guidelines. Table 13–1 provides some general advice for developing an initial treatment plan.

TABLE 13–1. Sequential ways to develop an initial treatment plan

1. Identify your patient's initial treatment goal.
2. Develop a therapeutic alliance with your patient.
3. Clarify the relationship between the caregiver and your patient.
4. Reach the most specific DSM-5 diagnosis for your patient.
5. Write a hierarchical list of current problems
6. Rewrite the problem list into treatment goals.
7. Identify measurable and achievable goals from the available evidence base.
8. Customize the treatment for your patient's cultural background and available resources.
9. Assign responsibility for each goal to a member of your patient's treatment team.
10. Monitor the progress toward each goal.
11. Revise the goals as your patient's situation changes.

Chapter 14

Psychosocial Interventions

When you assess and address a child or an adolescent's mental and behavioral health problems, you often direct caregivers to resources or interventions that they will deliver themselves. After all, most care for persons is delivered at home—where children are welcomed, fed, cleaned, taught, and nurtured. Motivated caregivers can implement evidence-supported care strategies that they learn from you or from handouts, books, Web sites, or videos you recommend. As noted in Chapter 2, "Addressing Behavioral and Mental Problems in Community Settings," such bibliotherapy has shown clinical effectiveness in some situations. Pediatric primary care practitioners tend to be particularly skilled in the realm of offering psychosocial intervention advice, because a key part of that professional role is offering parenting advice and anticipatory guidance.

This chapter contains selected highlights from among the psychosocial intervention strategies and tips we often describe for caregivers. Their inspiration comes from many different sources, including lessons from different lines of clinical research, general professional consensus, and personal experience (Chorpita and Daleiden 2009; Hilt 2014; Jellinek et al. 2002). This is not meant to be an exhaustive list of psychosocial strategies but rather a few we think you may find useful. These may be either sufficient on their own to resolve a mild concern or used to supplement specialist-delivered services.

Time-Out

Time-out is a strategy by which caregivers shape a young child's behavior through selective and temporary removal of that child's access to desired attention, activities, or other reinforcements following a behavioral transgression. This strategy works only for a child who experiences regular positive praise and attention from his caregiver because the child feels motivated to maintain that positive regard. The temporary removal of desired attention from a time-out can happen anywhere, not just via physically placing a child into a designated time-out area.

It is often said that the length of a time-out should be about 1 minute for each year of age, but adjustments need to be made on the basis of developmental level—for instance, time-outs for a developmentally delayed child should have shorter durations.

Although time-outs may be simple in concept, they are often difficult to implement. The following is a list of parent tips for time-out.

- To avoid confusion, set consistent limits.
- Focus on changing the priority misbehaviors rather than everything at once.
- After announcing time-out, decline further verbal engagement until "time-in."
- Ensure that time-outs occur immediately after misbehavior instead of being delayed.
- Follow through if using warnings (e.g., I'm going to count to three…).
- Minimize reinforcement of misbehavior with calm, quiet limit-setting.
- State when the time-out is over (the child does not determine this). Setting a timer may help.
- When the time-out finishes, simply "resume business as usual" or congratulate the child on regaining personal control. Then look for the next positive behavior to praise.
- For time-outs to help, give children far more positive attention than negative attention.

Special Time

Special time is a way for a caregiver and young child to reestablish the enjoyment of each other's company. Sometimes this reestablishment of positive caregiver-child interactions alone will be able to resolve a chronic behavior problem. Special time also can be referred to as *child-directed play* because it emphasizes that parents spend that time following their child's lead and attending to what the child can do. The following is a list of parent tips for successful use of special time.

- Commit to setting aside a regular time to try this with your child. Daily is best, but two to three times a week consistently also works.
- Select time of day, labeling it as something like *our play time* or *our special time*.
- Choose a time short enough that it can happen reliably, usually 15–30 minutes.
- Once this one-on-one time is planned, ensure that it happens no matter how good or bad the day was.
- Allow child to pick the together activity, which must be something you do not actively dislike and that does not involve spending money or completing a chore.
- Follow the child's lead during play, resisting urges to tell him or her what to do.
- End on time; a timer may help. Remind the child when the next special time will be.
- If the child refuses at first, explain that you will just sit with him for his special time.
- Expect greater success if you as a caregiver get your own special or nurturing times too.

Functional Analysis (of Behavior)

Functional analysis is a general strategy for resolving a recurrent problem behavior. Functional analysis is most often cited as a treatment for a child with developmental impairments or a limited verbal capacity, but its principles apply to any child. The objective is to first identify *why* a behavior keeps recurring and then intelligently devise a plan to prevent future repetitions.

For instance, imagine a young child throws tantrums during trips to stores. When a health care practitioner helps to analyze the behavior's function, the child's caregiver realizes he has been giving the child candy to halt the tantrums, which for the child functionally serves to reward the behavior and encourage it to happen again. If the caregiver chooses to stop delivering these unintentional rewards, the tantrum behavior would be theorized to decrease, although usually after a temporary increase in the behavior while the child tests out the new rules (an *extinction burst*). Alternatively, a caregiver may focus on avoiding reexposing the child to a recognized behavior trigger, such as no longer bringing the child into a store's candy aisle. The following is a list of tips for performing a functional analysis of behavior (Hanley et al. 2003; Hilt 2014).

1. Identify the behavior.

   - Determine the character, timing (especially what happens before and after), frequency, and duration of the behavior.

2. Analyze and hypothesize about the behavior's function.

   - Achieve a goal. This might include escaping an undesired situation, avoiding a transition, acquiring attention, or getting access to desired things.
   - Communicate. Maladaptive behavior may communicate physical or emotional discomfort.
   - If no function is clear, other causes such as medical or psychiatric disorders, medication side effects, and sleep deprivation become more likely.

3. Make a change, usually changing something in the environment.

   - Remove future reinforcements for the maladaptive behavior (attention or other gains).
   - Avoid known behavioral triggers.
   - Modify task demands to be appropriate for developmental stage and language ability.
   - Reinforce positive behaviors with attention and praise.
   - Enhance communication (e.g., helping a nonverbal child use pictures to communicate).
   - Clarify any unclear expectations—show or follow a daily schedule; prepare a child for transitions.
   - Allow child access to escapes when overwhelmed (time limited in a calm, quiet place).

4. Analyze if the interventions worked, and if not, repeat the process.

   - Look for improvements in the behavior's timing, character, frequency, and duration.

Behavioral Activation

Behavioral activation is a way to help a young person reengage with other people. When a young person is sad or worried, he is less likely to engage in the activities he typically enjoys, and this withdrawal from otherwise pleasurable activities deepens his isolation and lowers mood. Therefore, despite other areas of difference, most cognitive-behavioral therapies for depression and anxiety will seek behavioral activation. After all, the path to recovery from depression and anxiety does not begin with spending all your time alone in a darkened room.

In behavioral activation, a person pushes himself to more regularly do things that he finds pleasurable or that serve his goals. If he can accomplish this behavioral activation, his symptoms usually will improve. The challenge is to create the necessary motivation when feeling depressed or anxious. The following is a list of tips for succeeding with behavioral activation.

- Identify activities that you (not others) would find motivating or rewarding. Work on developing a variety of options because repetitively doing the same thing can get boring.
- Refine the list to things that can be measured as completed rather than relatively vague goals that you cannot determine whether they are completed.
- Rank the activities in order from those that would be easier to those that would be more difficult to complete.
- Start by selecting something easy to accomplish to get started and work your way up the list from there.
- Let others know your plans to increase your activities and enlist their help in motivating you further.

Bullying: Dealing With a Common Problem

For years, it has been recognized that bullying is both common and harmful for both the victim and the perpetrator. If you notice a relatively sudden change in a child's mood, behavior, sleep, or body symptoms or any sudden change in social or academic functioning, then you should consider the possibility he is being bullied.

If bullying is discovered, it is often challenging for an adult to know how to respond. The following is a list of tips for how to respond to bullying (Buxton et al. 2013; Hilt 2014).

1. Detect
   - Ask the child: "I know kids sometimes get picked on or bullied. Have you ever seen this happen? Has this ever happened to you?"

- If the child says no, but you still suspect bullying, have caregivers ask teachers about bullying and/or review the child's social media accounts.

2. Educate
   - Let children know that bullying is unacceptable and that if they encounter bullying, you will help them respond.

3. Plan
   - Coach the child to avoid places where bullying happens.
   - Teach the child to walk away when bullying occurs and tell a trusted adult who can be accessed quickly.
   - Instruct the child to stay near adults—most bullying happens when no adults are around.
   - If a child feels that he can confront the bully, teach him to say, in a calm, clear voice, to stop the behavior, that "bullying is not OK."
   - Note that if a child is comfortable with deflating situations with humor, he may use humor to challenge the bullying.
   - Encourage a child to ask his peers for their support and ideas.
   - Ensure that caregivers communicate the problem to a child's school and other families, jointly devising solutions.

4. Support
   - Tell caregivers to encourage participation in prosocial activities to build peer networks, enhance social skills, and gain confidence. Additional information is available on Web sites such as www.stopbullying.gov.

Sleep Hygiene

Sleep hygiene is a good idea for anyone, but especially for young people. Insomnia is a common problem among children and adolescents. Most sleep problems can be resolved by changing habits and routines that affect sleep, what practitioners call good sleep hygiene. The following is a list of parent tips for how to improve sleep hygiene (Hilt 2014; Mindell and Owens 2009).

- Maintain consistent bedtimes and wake times every day of the week.
- Maintain a routine of presleep activities (e.g., read a book, brush teeth).
- Avoid spending nonsleep time in or on one's bed (i.e., "beds are for sleep").
- Ensure that the bedroom is cool and quiet.
- Avoid high-stimulation activities just before bed or during awakenings (television, video games, texting friends, or exercise).
- Do not keep video games, televisions, computers, or phones in a child's bedroom.
- Do physical exercise earlier in the day to help with sleep hours later.
- Avoid caffeine in the afternoons and evenings, which can cause shallow sleep or frequent awakenings.
- If awake in bed and unable to sleep, get out of bed for a low-stimulation activity, (e.g., reading), then return 20–30 minutes later. This keeps the bed from becoming associated with sleeplessness.
- Encourage children and adolescents to discuss any worries with a caregiver before bed rather than ruminating later.
- Ensure that children go to bed drowsy but still awake. Falling asleep in other places forms habits that are difficult to break.
- Use security objects at bedtime for a young child who needs a transitional object with which to feel safe and secure when his caregiver is not present.
- When checking on a young child at night, aim to only briefly reassure the child that you are present and that he is OK.
- Avoid afternoon naps for all but the very young because they often interfere with nighttime sleep.
- If a child or an adolescent is still having difficulties, keep a sleep diary to help you track his naps, sleep times, and activities to identify patterns.

Postcrisis Planning for Caregivers

From time to time, major crisis events happen with young people. This might involve a major argument, an emotional trauma, or a child threatening to hurt himself. The first steps are to address any acute safety concerns and obtain any necessary professional assistance. Afterward, it can be helpful to develop a prevention plan for future crises. The following is a list of parent tips for postcrisis planning in the home.

1. In the home environment, maintain a "low-key" atmosphere and keep up regular routines.
2. Follow typical house rules, but pick your battles; for example:

   • If a child engages in aggressive or dangerous behaviors, intervene immediately.
   • If a child is using oppositional words, you may be able to ignore those words.

3. Provide appropriate supervision until the crisis is resolved (i.e., always have an adult around).
4. Make a specific crisis prevention plan:

   • Identify likely triggers for a crisis (such as an argument).
   • Plan with the child what to do the next time the triggers occur (e.g., remove self from the situation until feeling calm again, call a friend, engage in a distracting activity).

5. Encourage your child to attend school, unless otherwise directed by a practitioner.
6. Attend the next scheduled appointment with your practitioner.
7. Administer medications as directed by the child's medical or psychiatric practitioner.
8. Enter into each day and evening with a plan for how time will be spent—this should help prevent boredom and arguments in the moment.
9. If there are self-harm risks, secure and lock up all medications and objects a child or an adolescent could use to hurt himself, including

   • Sharp objects such as knives and razors
   • Materials that can be used for strangulation attempts, such as belts, cords, ropes, and sheets
   • Firearms and ammunition (locked and kept in separate locations from each other)
   • Medications of all family members, including all over-the-counter medicines

10. In the event of another crisis,
    - Contact your health care provider.
    - Call 911 to have your child transported to the nearest emergency department if you believe that he, yourself, or another person is no longer safe as a result of his behavior.
    - Consider using local and national crisis and suicide hotlines.

Chapter 15

Psychotherapeutic Interventions

The most effective treatment plan for any young person with a mental disorder will include some form of psychotherapy. At the very least, any treatment plan will include the formation of a therapeutic alliance with you as the care practitioner and psychoeducation about diagnosis, treatment, and prognosis. Several evidence-based textbooks teach more advanced psychotherapy techniques for working with children and adolescents (e.g., Christophersen and VanScoyoc 2013; Kendall 2012; Weisz and Kazdin 2010). These psychotherapy skills are typically learned during training programs when senior practitioners supervise trainees. Although we recommend these texts and psychotherapy training to everyone who regularly works with children and adolescents, in this chapter we introduce different kinds of psychotherapy, discuss how to select a particular psychotherapy, and explain how to engage a child and her caregivers in psychotherapy.

Psychotherapy is an important treatment strategy for young people for many reasons. It is almost always the safest treatment option we can offer and has the least potential for adverse effects. For specific problems, such as disruptive behavior or suicidality, it also has shown superior efficacy over psychotropic medication interventions. In addition, the psychotherapeutic literature has shown that when a person attributes a behavioral change to her own efforts, the change is more enduring than a behavioral change she attributes to an external source, such as a medication (Alarcón and Frank 2011).

However, the changes that result from psychotherapy generally are not immediate—we expect it to take a month or two of regular sessions before a child or an adolescent begins to manifest the benefits of psychotherapy. This delay is part of the reason why it is important to stratify the severity of a young person's mental distress. If a child or an adolescent is having moderate to severe difficulties, our preferred treatment plan is more likely to include a combination of both psychotherapy and medication to encourage the most rapid and reliable results. For young people who have a mild degree of mental health difficulties, our treatment plans typically begin with psychotherapy alone. Of course, these are broad generalizations, and many exceptions exist. For instance, even with severe oppositional defiant disorder, we prefer to start treatment with behavioral management training instead of psychotropic medications. In contrast, it is clinically reasonable to initiate treatment for severe attention-deficit/hyperactivity disorder with stimulant medications alone.

If you decide to recommend psychotherapy, it can be difficult to know which psychotherapy to recommend because there are a large (and growing) number of different validated psychotherapies that can be delivered to children. For example, on its Web site (www.nrepp.samhsa.gov), the U.S. Substance Abuse and Mental Health Services Administration lists more than 200 different research evidence–based psychotherapies for young people. Fortunately, even though these therapies have significant differences, they are often variations on a small number of themes. For example, TF-CBT seems like a confusing acronym, but it is actually a trauma-focused version of cognitive-behavioral therapy, a widely practiced evidence-based psychotherapy.

Even after you identify the appropriate psychotherapy for a particular child or adolescent, it can be difficult to engage a young person and her caregivers in the therapy. In meta-analyses, between 25% and 75% of children and adolescents in mental health treatment prematurely discontinue (de Haan et al. 2013), a finding that illustrates the challenges of delivering treatment. Engagement in psychotherapy can be a barrier because of stigma, ambivalence about behavior change, doubts about the efficacy of psychotherapy, the time investment it requires, or financial barriers. You can help by communicating appropriate expectations for psychotherapy with a patient and her caregivers, informing them of the efficacy of psychotherapy, the delayed response, and its enduring benefits.

How else can you engage a patient and her caregivers in psychotherapy?

- Explain the diagnosis in a way that the patient and her caregivers can fully understand.

- Explain the rationale for the psychotherapy treatment plan (e.g., as the safest or most effective approach).
- Briefly describe what the recommended psychotherapy experience would be like.
- Ask if they have any concerns about that approach in order to address them.
- Provide the family with a list of recommended practitioners.
- Follow up with the family to address any problems that arise.

This last follow-up step in particular is important because families often get discouraged if they run into an insurance coverage restriction or have trouble finding an available practitioner. Discussing what happened with the referral provides you an opportunity to amend the care plan. In general, referrals are most successful when you can match a patient and her caregiver with a therapist with whom they form a therapeutic alliance (Roos and Werbart 2013).

After all, the heart of all psychiatric treatments is the therapeutic alliance you establish when a patient identifies treatment goals and you ally yourself with the patient as she pursues those goals. You form an alliance between yourself and your patient with the goal of mobilizing healing forces within your patient by psychological means. Your ability to form these alliances profoundly influences the efficacy of your work for the patient, as well as your satisfaction with this work (Summers and Barber 2003).

To assist you, we prepared descriptions of different types of psychotherapy that are commonly considered with children and adolescents and a list of conditions for which their use has been validated as effective by research (Table 15–1).

TABLE 15–1. Commonly recommended child and adolescent psychotherapies

Therapy	General description	Typical indications
Cognitive-behavioral therapy (CBT)	Teaches patients how to correct illness-related cognitive errors in thinking (e.g., the depressed patient thinking "nothing ever goes right for me") and coaches/encourages patients to try out different behaviors (i.e., behavior activation)—both of which lead to changes in how the person feels. Assigning practice and trials between sessions is a core feature. Desensitization via supported exposure to one's fears is typically used for anxiety.	Anxiety disorders (all) Depressive disorders Oppositional defiant disorder Eating disorders Substance use disorders Posttraumatic stress disorder
Trauma-focused CBT	Most commonly cited version of trauma therapy in children. Starts with building therapeutic support and educating about posttraumatic stress disorder. Like other successful trauma therapies, treatment requires patients to face their own trauma narrative to desensitize, reduce pathological avoidance, and reduce the trauma memory's control over their future.	

TABLE 15–1. Commonly recommended child and adolescent psychotherapies (*continued*)

Therapy	General description	Typical indications
Dialectical behavior therapy	Very specialized version of CBT; requires attending skills groups (to teach problem solving, emotional regulation, distress tolerance, and interpersonal effectiveness skills) and attending individual therapy sessions. Mindfulness and meditative exercises are often used to assist. Uniquely helpful for treatment-resistant, chronically suicidal patients. Most supportive research is with adults.	Chronic and significant suicidality and self-harm
Family therapy	Many different styles and approaches, but all focus on the family relationship or interaction patterns that cause dysfunction and help the family system to amend that pattern (rather than identifying a mental health diagnosis to treat or saying that the problem resides within an individual).	Eating disorders Conduct disorder Depressive disorders Substance use disorders
Group therapy	Addresses interaction pattern problems, as in family therapy, while providing more disorder-specific support within a group of strangers having similar challenges. Peer-based learning can be uniquely effective. Therapists must steer group members away from inadvertently teaching unhealthy behaviors.	Anxiety disorders

TABLE 15–1. Commonly recommended child and adolescent psychotherapies *(continued)*

Therapy	General description	Typical indications
Behavior management training	General term for programs that teach and encourage skillful parent or caregiver responses to challenging child behaviors. Positive interaction time between the parent and the child is encouraged because it must accompany behavioral management steps in order to work. Changing caregiver behaviors is key rather than changing the child through individual therapy sessions. Also known as parent management training.	Oppositional defiant disorder Conduct disorder
Applied behavioral analysis	One-on-one specialized intensive behavioral management training that gradually teaches socially normative behaviors via small achievable elements, with each element reinforced by a reward (such as rewarding the child making any "h" sound as step in teaching use of "hello"). Highly resource intensive in terms of the required therapist hours and continuous treatment planning.	Autism spectrum disorder

TABLE 15–1. Commonly recommended child and adolescent psychotherapies (*continued*)

Therapy	General description	Typical indications
Social skills training	Variety of class-based, group, and one-to-one techniques to teach basic behavioral and cognitive skills, reinforce prosocial behaviors, and teach social problem solving. More potent when delivered in a group rather than a one-to-one setting because of peer learning influences.	Oppositional defiant disorder Attention-deficit/ hyperactivity disorder Autism spectrum disorder
Relaxation training	Biofeedback, deep breathing, progressive muscle relaxation, and mindfulness are examples of strategies used to increase mind-body awareness and the ability to electively calm the heights of emotional reactions. Must be practiced when not in crisis in order to develop the skills needed for times of crisis.	Anxiety disorders Depressive disorders
Motivational interviewing	Therapeutic interaction regarding health behavior(s) around which a patient needs to change but has significant reluctance. Nonconfrontationally and nonjudgmentally helps patients to state their own reasons for changing, to resolve their own ambivalence, and to state what actions they could take to change. Most supportive research is with adults.	Substance use disorders

Chapter 16

Psychopharmacological Interventions

As the efficacy of psychotropic medications has been demonstrated by research and their use destigmatized, their prescription to children and adolescents has become commonplace. For example, when adolescents in the United States were recently surveyed, more than 6% reported using a psychotropic medication in the past month (Jonas et al. 2013). This relatively widespread use of psychotropic medications means that caregivers have come to expect primary care practitioners, not just mental health specialists, to consider prescribing medication for a child or an adolescent with a mental illness.

When should a psychotropic medication be prescribed? Not every child with depression, anxiety, or attention-deficit/hyperactivity disorder (ADHD) needs to receive a medication, regardless of whether it fits an approved or research-supported indication. Because psychiatric medications can cause adverse effects, you must, at a minimum, believe that the potential benefit of psychotropic medication exceeds the potential risks your patient may experience. For instance, if a child has a relatively mild case of depression, psychotherapy alone is usually sufficient to help, and its use does not introduce the risk of medical adverse effects. If a child or an adolescent's depression is more severe or persistent, use of a selective serotonin reuptake inhibitor (SSRI) combined with psychotherapy makes better clinical sense to achieve a more rapid recovery (e.g., Emslie et al. 2010).

As a rule of thumb, if a child or an adolescent has a moderate to severe range of symptoms and an evidence-based psychotropic medication is available, we usually prescribe the medication at the same time we initiate the appropriate psychosocial interventions. For a child or an adolescent with milder symptoms, we generally recommend starting treatment with psychotherapy or environmental interventions alone. Those with mild symptoms but persistent dysfunction become stronger candidates for a medication treatment when nonmedication strategies prove to be ineffective.

When approaching the decision about what to prescribe, we advise following evidence-based principles. Although we appreciate the wisdom of experienced practitioners and the insights reported in case series, these are small, unstandardized accounts. Whenever possible, we base our prescribing decisions on evidence generated from controlled trials conducted among children and adolescents. For practitioners who frequently prescribe psychotropic medications to children and adolescents, we recommend reading the evidence-based systematic reviews published by the *Cochrane Database of Systematic Reviews,* the Practice Parameters published by the American Academy of Child and Adolescent Psychiatry, or one of the available textbooks (e.g., McVoy and Findling 2013; Preston et al. 2015).

When such evidence is unavailable, we find that adult mental health medication research is informative but in need of translation before we can use the medication for children and adolescents. Children and adolescents are not "little adults" who will respond to "little doses" in the same way that adults do. For example, tricyclic antidepressants are effective in the treatment of depression in adults, but controlled trials found that tricyclic antidepressants are no better than placebo in the treatment of depression in children and are of marginal utility for treating depression in adolescents (Hazell and Mirzaie 2013). A result from the adult mental health literature therefore must be replicated in children and adolescents before it can be reliably followed.

However, appropriate evidence-based care does not mean limiting your prescriptions to only those medications approved for children and adolescents by a regulatory agency such as the U.S. Food and Drug Administration (FDA). Pediatric approvals exist for only about half of all the medications used with children, such that nearly three-fourths of all hospital-delivered medications (both medical and psychiatric) lack an age-matched pediatric regulatory approval (Murthy et al. 2013). This regulatory discrepancy occurs largely because the process of obtaining an FDA approval is a long and expensive endeavor that requires a vested party (the manufacturer). Rigorous research may support the use of medication without such an approval.

Some of the key questions we ask ourselves before prescribing any medication include the following:

- Diagnosis—does the child have an evidence-based medication indication?
- Age—how does the child's age change your risk-benefit analysis?
- Severity—how rapid of a treatment response is needed?
- History—what has already been tried, and how effective was it?
- Preferences—are there strong patient or caregiver opinions about the use of medication?

Practitioners may feel pressured to use medications well outside of evidence-based indications when patients and caregivers are struggling. We prefer to resist these demands and limit the prescription of psychotropic medications to the indications for which sound evidence exists. For instance, prescribing methylphenidate for a child whose poor school performance is not due to ADHD but rather is due to a learning disability, anxiety, social distractions, or depression may be ineffective and delay the use of more appropriate interventions. Similarly, antipsychotics may reduce the severity of nonspecific aggression, but they are unlikely to address the underlying causes of youth aggression and may unnecessarily introduce major adverse effects.

Tables 16–1 to 16–5 include only those psychotropic medications with a randomized controlled trial evidence base for use with young people. The age ranges of the listed FDA approvals do not necessarily reflect the age ranges for which these medications are clinically appropriate or effective.

Older antipsychotic medications with long-standing FDA approvals for use in young people include haloperidol (≥3 years old) for severe aggression and Tourette's disorder, pimozide (≥12 years old) for Tourette's disorder, chlorpromazine (≥1 year old) for severe aggression, and thioridazine (≥ 2 years old) for schizophrenia. However, concern about adverse effects, chiefly movement disorders, limits contemporary use of these medications in children and adolescents.

Psychopharmacological Monitoring for Adverse Effects

When we prescribe a medication to a child or an adolescent, we take responsibility for monitoring for the development of

TABLE 16–1. Attention-deficit/hyperactivity disorder: short-acting evidence-based stimulant medications

Drug name	Stimulant class	Duration (hours)	Usual 6- to 10-year-old starting doses	Available doses (mg tablets)	FDA maximum daily dose (mg; approval ages)	Editorial comments
Methylphenidate (Ritalin, Methylin)	Methylphenidate	4–6	5 mg bid (2.5 mg if 3–5 years)	5, 10, 20	60 (≥6)	May have fewer side effects than dextroamphetamine; better evidence for very young children

TABLE 16–1. Attention-deficit/hyperactivity disorder: short-acting evidence-based stimulant medications *(continued)*

Drug name	Stimulant class	Duration (hours)	Usual 6- to 10-year-old starting doses	Available doses (mg tablets)	FDA maximum daily dose (mg; approval ages)	Editorial comments
Dexmethylphenidate (Focalin)	Methylphenidate	4–6	2.5 mg bid (1.25 mg if 3–5 years)	2.5, 5, 10	20 (≥6)	Racemic isomer, so has twice the mg:mg potency of methylphenidate
Dextroamphetamine (Dexedrine, DextroStat)	Dextroamphetamine	4–6	2.5 mg bid (1.25 mg if 3–5 years)	2.5, 5, 7.5, 10, 20, 30	40 (≥3)	Tends to have longer duration than methylphenidate; slightly more side effects

TABLE 16–1. Attention-deficit/hyperactivity disorder: short-acting evidence-based stimulant medications (*continued*)

Drug name	Stimulant class	Duration (hours)	Usual 6- to 10-year-old starting doses	Available doses (mg tablets)	FDA maximum daily dose (mg; approval ages)	Editorial comments
Amphetamine salt combination (Adderall)	Dextroamphetamine	4–6	2.5 mg bid (1.25 mg if 3–5 years)	5, 7.5, 10, 12.5, 15, 20, 30	40 (≥3)	Tends to have longer duration than methylphenidate; slightly more side effects

Note. bid = twice a day; FDA = U.S. Food and Drug Administration.

TABLE 16–2. Attention-deficit/hyperactivity disorder: long-acting evidence-based stimulant medications

Drug name	Stimulant class	Duration (hours)	Usual 6- to 10-year-old starting doses (mg)	Available doses	FDA maximum daily dose (mg; approval ages)	Editorial comments
Methylphenidate ER/SR (Metadate ER)	Methylphenidate	4–8	10 qam	10, 20 mg tablets	60 (≥6)	Uses a wax matrix for delivery; variable duration of action
OROS methylphenidate (Concerta)	Methylphenidate	10–12	18 qam	18, 27, 36, 54 mg capsules	72 (≥6)	Osmotic release capsule; cannot be cut or crushed
Methylphenidate XR oral suspension (Quillivant XR)	Methylphenidate	Up to 8	20 qam	5 mg/mL liquid	60 (≥6)	Microsuspension yields an ER liquid

TABLE 16–2. Attention-deficit/hyperactivity disorder: long-acting evidence-based stimulant medications (*continued*)

Drug name	Stimulant class	Duration (hours)	Usual 6- to 10-year-old starting doses (mg)	Available doses	FDA maximum daily dose (mg; approval ages)	Editorial comments
Methylphenidate XR; 30% IR, 70% ER (Metadate CD)	Methylphenidate	~8	10 qam	10, 20, 30, 40, 50, 60 mg capsules	60 (≥6)	Beads in capsule can be sprinkled on food
Methylphenidate XR; 50% IR, 50% ER (Ritalin LA)	Methylphenidate	~8	10 qam	10, 20, 30, 40 mg capsules	60 (≥6)	Beads in capsule can be sprinkled on food
Dexmethylphenidate XR (Focalin XR)	Methylphenidate	10–12	5 qam	5, 10, 15, 20 mg capsules	30 (≥6)	Beads in capsule are a racemic isomer of methylphenidate, so this medication has twice the mg potency

TABLE 16–2. Attention-deficit/hyperactivity disorder: long-acting evidence-based stimulant medications *(continued)*

Drug name	Stimulant class	Duration (hours)	Usual 6- to 10-year-old starting doses (mg)	Available doses	FDA maximum daily dose (mg; approval ages)	Editorial comments
Methylphenidate patch (Daytrana)	Methylphenidate	Until 3–5 hours after patch removal	10 qam	10, 15, 20, 30 mg patch	30 (≥6)	Site rash problems; slow morning startup of effects; works until removed
Amphetamine salt combo-XR (Adderall XR)	Dextroamphetamine	8–12	5 qd	5, 10, 15, 20, 25, 30 mg capsules	30 (≥6)	Generic available; beads in capsule can be sprinkled on food

TABLE 16–2. Attention-deficit/hyperactivity disorder: long-acting evidence-based stimulant medications (*continued*)

Drug name	Stimulant class	Duration (hours)	Usual 6- to 10-year-old starting doses (mg)	Available doses	FDA maximum daily dose (mg; approval ages)	Editorial comments
Lisdexamfetamine (Vyvanse)	Dextroamphet-amine	~10	30 qd	20, 30, 40, 50, 60, 70 mg capsules	70 (≥6)	Conversion ratio from dextroamphetamine not well established; gastrointestinal bioactivation
Dextroamphetamine ER (Dexedrine Spansule)	Dextroamphet-amine	8–10	5 qam	5, 10, 15 mg capsules	40 (≥6)	Beads in capsule can be sprinkled on food

Note. bid=twice a day; ER=extended release; FDA=U.S. Food and Drug Administration; IR=immediate release; OROS=osmotic controlled-release oral delivery system; qam=every morning; qd=every day; SR=sustained release; XR=extended release.

TABLE 16–3. Attention-deficit/hyperactivity disorder (ADHD): nonstimulant evidence-based medications

Drug name	Half-life (hours)	Medication type	Usual starting doses	Available doses (mg)	FDA maximum daily dose (approval ages)	Editorial comments
Atomoxetine (Strattera)	5	Norepinephrine reuptake inhibitor	0.5 mg/kg once a day then 1.2 mg/kg/day after 1 week	10, 18, 25, 40, 60, 80, 100 capsules	100 mg or 1.4 mg/kg/day, whichever is less (≥6)	Side effect risks same as with SSRIs (e.g., suicidality warning); cytochrome P450 2D6 metabolism; about 50% respond
Clonidine (Catapres)	12.5	Central-acting α_2-agonist	0.05 mg bid	0.1, 0.2, 0.3, 0.4 tablets	0.4 mg	Dosing at bedtime may help manage sedation effects

TABLE 16–3. Attention-deficit/hyperactivity disorder (ADHD): nonstimulant evidence-based medications *(continued)*

Drug name	Half-life (hours)	Medication type	Usual starting doses	Available doses (mg)	FDA maximum daily dose (approval ages)	Editorial comments
Clonidine XR (Kapvay)	12.5	Central-acting α_2-agonist	0.1 mg qd	0.1, 0.2, 0.3, 0.4 tablets	0.4 mg ($\geq$6)	Difference is a reduced peak blood level relative to IR form
Guanfacine (Tenex)	16	Central-acting α_2-agonist	1 mg qd	1, 2, 3, 4 tablets	4 mg	Dosing at bedtime may help manage sedation effects
Guanfacine XR (Intuniv)	18	Central-acting α_2-agonist	1 mg qd	0.1, 0.2, 0.3, 0.4 tablets	7 mg ($\geq$6)	Difference is a reduced peak blood level relative to IR form

Note. bid=twice a day; FDA=U.S. Food and Drug Administration; IR=immediate release; qd=every day; SSRIs=selective serotonin reuptake inhibitors; XR=extended release. Unlike stimulants, these medications may take up to a month to generate their full efficacy in the treatment of ADHD in children and adolescents. Stimulants are considered the first-line treatment option.

TABLE 16–4. Depressive and anxiety disorders: evidence-based medications

Drug name	Half-life	Usual teenage starting dose (mg)	FDA maximum daily dose (approval ages)	Available doses	Conditions with RCT support	Editorial comments
Fluoxetine (Prozac)	4–6 days	10 qam	60 mg (≥7 OCD, ≥8 MDD)	10, 20, 40 mg capsules	OCD, MDD, GAD, SAD, SOC	First-line treatment for both depression and anxiety; long half-life reduces side effects from missed doses
Sertraline (Zoloft)	27 hours	50 qam	200 mg (≥6 OCD)	25, 50, 100 mg tablets	OCD, MDD, GAD, SAD, SOC	First-line treatment for anxiety; easy to use small doses (i.e., half of a 25 mg tab)
Citalopram (Celexa)	35 hours	20 qam	40 mg in adults (not child approved)	10, 20, 40 mg tablets	MDD, OCD	Very few drug-drug interactions

TABLE 16–4. Depressive and anxiety disorders: evidence-based medications *(continued)*

Drug name	Half-life	Usual teenage starting dose (mg)	FDA maximum daily dose (approval ages)	Available doses	Conditions with RCT support	Editorial comments
Escitalopram (Lexapro)	29.5 hours	10 qam	20 mg (≥12 MDD)	5, 10, 20 mg tablets	MDD	Racemic isomer of citalopram; very few drug-drug interactions
Fluvoxamine (Luvox)	16 hours	25 qam	300 mg (≥8 OCD)	25, 50, 100 mg tablets	OCD, GAD, SOC, SAD	Often more side effects than other SSRIs; many drug-drug interactions; thus, not a first-line option
Paroxetine (Paxil)	18 hours	20 qam	40 mg in adults (not child approved)	10, 20, 30, 40 mg tablets	SOC	Mixed evidence; not preferred for child depression

TABLE 16–4. Depressive and anxiety disorders: evidence-based medications (*continued*)

Drug name	Half-life	Usual teenage starting dose (mg)	FDA maximum daily dose (approval ages)	Available doses	Conditions with RCT support	Editorial comments
Clomipramine (Anafranil)	32 hours	25 mg	200 mg or 3 mg/kg/day (≥10 OCD)	25, 50, 75 mg capsules	OCD	Tricyclic, used for treatment-resistant OCD; not a first-line option because of greater adverse effects than with SSRIs
Duloxetine (Cymbalta)	12 hours	30 qd	120 mg (≥7 GAD)	20, 30, 60 mg capsules	GAD	Serotonin-norepinephrine reuptake inhibitor; has more adverse effects than SSRIs

Note. FDA=U.S. Food and Drug Administration; GAD=generalized anxiety disorder; MDD=major depressive disorder; OCD=obsessive-compulsive disorder; qam=every morning; qd=every day; RCT=randomized controlled trial; SAD=separation anxiety disorder; SOC=social phobia; SSRIs=selective serotonin reuptake inhibitors.

TABLE 16–5. Bipolar and psychotic disorders: evidence-based medications

Drug name	Half-life (hours)	Usual teenage starting dose (mg)	FDA maximum daily dose (approval ages)	Available doses (mg)	Conditions with RCT support	Editorial comments
Risperidone (Risperdal)	17	0.5 qd	6 mg (≥13 schizophrenia, ≥10 bipolar mania, ≥5 autism irritability)	0.25, 0.5, 1, 2, 3, 4 tablets	Schizophrenia, bipolar mania, autism, Tourette's disorder	Extensively studied in children; has relatively consistent and rapid effects; extra risk of prolactinemia
Aripiprazole (Abilify)	75	2 qd	30 mg (≥13 schizophrenia, ≥10 bipolar mania, ≥6 autism irritability, ≥6 Tourette's disorder)	2, 5, 10, 15, 20 tablets	Schizophrenia, bipolar mania, autism, Tourette's disorder	Mixed agonist/antagonist at dopamine D$_2$ receptor; may cause irritability; takes longer than others to see clinical changes

TABLE 16–5. Bipolar and psychotic disorders: evidence-based medications (*continued*)

Drug name	Half-life (hours)	Usual teenage starting dose (mg)	FDA maximum daily dose (approval ages)	Available doses (mg)	Conditions with RCT support	Editorial comments
Quetiapine (Seroquel)	7	25 bid	800 mg (≥13 schizophrenia, ≥10 bipolar mania)	25, 50, 100, 200, 300, 400 tablets	Schizophrenia, bipolar mania	Pills larger so might be harder to swallow; noted anxiolytic properties
Ziprasidone (Geodon)	7	10 qam	160 mg/day in adults (not child approved)	20, 40, 60, 80 capsules	Schizophrenia, bipolar mania	Greater risk of QT lengthening, so electrocardiogram monitoring is necessary; not a first-line option for children

TABLE 16–5. Bipolar and psychotic disorders: evidence-based medications *(continued)*

Drug name	Half-life (hours)	Usual teenage starting dose (mg)	FDA maximum daily dose (approval ages)	Available doses (mg)	Conditions with RCT support	Editorial comments
Olanzapine (Zyprexa)	30	2.5 qam	20 mg (≥13 schizophrenia, ≥13 bipolar mania, ≥10 bipolar depression, with fluoxetine)	2.5, 5, 7.5, 10, 15, 20 tablets	Schizophrenia, bipolar mania, bipolar depression	Has rapid benefits but greatest risk of weight gain and lipid changes in this group
Paliperidone (Invega)	23	3 qd	12 mg (≥12 schizophrenia)	1.5, 3, 6, 9 tablets	Schizophrenia	Major active metabolite of risperidone; similar risk of hyperprolactinemia

Note. bid=twice a day; FDA=U.S. Food and Drug Administration; qd=every day.

known adverse effects. The tables in the following subsections are drawn from the published literature (Hilt 2012) and from adverse effect labeling from medication manufacturers (U.S. Food and Drug Administration 2015).

Stimulants

Stimulants (i.e., methylphenidate, dextroamphetamine) are usually well tolerated, but they often cause decreased appetite and insomnia (Table 16–6). Dose and duration of action adjustments typically mitigate these problems. Tracking growth on a growth curve greatly helps with recognizing weight gain problems (Table 16–7). Sometimes stimulants cause irritability or dysphoria, which may resolve by switching to the other family of stimulant. Excessive doses can cause cognitive dulling. Stimulants often cause a very slight elevation in heart rate or blood pressure that is almost always clinically insignificant, but we screen for outlier responses via a vital signs check after initiation. A tic disorder is no longer considered a contraindication for stimulant use because tics are just as likely to increase or decrease temporarily during stimulant use (Pringsheim and Steeves 2011).

Selective Serotonin Reuptake Inhibitors

Common SSRI side effects include a change in appetite that can lead to weight gain or loss and a sleep change that may include dreams becoming more vivid (Table 16–8). Diminished sex drive is common, although this problem is less notable for adolescents than for adults. Because platelets use serotonin for aggregation signaling, easier bruising may occur. Very high SSRI doses or combining serotonin agents could result in serotonin syndrome, which includes agitation, ataxia, diarrhea, hyperreflexia, mental status changes, tremor, and hyperthermia. Manic symptoms occur rarely as an SSRI side effect; this occurrence is not proof that the child will develop bipolar disorder. SSRIs have a common risk of causing irritability or agitation, which, if added to significant anxiety or depression might be a reason why there is a reported twofold elevation of self harm thoughts early in treatment when youth use SSRIs versus a placebo. Prescribers need to discuss this black box suicidality warning with patients and caregivers when prescribing a SSRI, along with the need for early treatment monitoring. Safe SSRI use involves examining a patient for adverse effects at around 2 weeks and

TABLE 16–6. Highlights of stimulant adverse effects

Common

Decreased appetite

Nausea

Weight loss

Insomnia

Headaches

Stomachaches

Dry mouth

Less common

Irritability

Dysphoria

Cognitive dulling

Obsessiveness

Anxiety

Tics

Dizziness

Blood pressure and pulse rate elevation

Notable rare reactions

Seizure

Hallucinations

Mania

Loss of adult height potential

TABLE 16–7. Monitoring suggestions for stimulants

Record height and weight growth curve at baseline and at each follow-up, at least every 6 months.

Measure blood pressure and pulse rate at baseline and after initiation of medication.

Monitor refill dates to identify signs of drug diversion.

Repeat administration of attention-deficit/hyperactivity disorder symptom rating scale until remission is achieved.

TABLE 16–8. Highlights of selective serotonin reuptake inhibitor adverse effects

Common

Insomnia

Sedation

Appetite increase

Appetite decrease

Nausea

Dry mouth

Headache

Sexual dysfunction

Less common

Agitation

Restlessness

Impulsivity

Irritability

Silliness

Dizziness

Tremor

Constipation

Diarrhea

Notable rare reactions

Suicidal thoughts

Serotonin syndrome

Easy bleeding

Hyponatremia

Mania

Prolonged QT interval

TABLE 16–9. Monitoring suggestions for selective serotonin reuptake inhibitors

Record height and weight at baseline and at each follow-up, at least every 6 months.

Inquire about increased irritability or agitation at 2 weeks and at 4–6 weeks after initiation.

Inquire about new or worsened suicidal thoughts at 2 weeks and at 4–6 weeks after initiation.

Inquire about new bleeding or bruising at least once after initiation.

Repeat disorder-specific rating scale(s) until remission is achieved. Takes 4–6 weeks to see benefits from a given dose.

again at 4–6 weeks after initiation to screen for worsening mood or irritability (Table 16–9) (Bridge et al. 2007).

Newer-Generation Antipsychotics

Antipsychotics for children and adolescents are typically initiated by mental health specialists, but primary care practitioners often find themselves in the role of providing refills or monitoring. Patients can experience fairly significant adverse effects from these medications (Table 16–10). Weight gain is the most common problem, with patients in some trials gaining an average of more than 10 pounds in just 3 months of medication use (Correll et al. 2009). Weight gain seems to occur more frequently in children than in adults—for instance, aripiprazole and risperidone have been found to cause equal degrees of weight gain in children, a finding that contradicts the adult literature (Correll et al. 2009). Muscle stiffness or dystonia may occur, particularly during initial use, for which practitioners can warn a family to keep diphenhydramine around as an antidote. Sedation is common, but this might be managed through bedtime dosing. A metabolic syndrome of elevated levels of blood glucose, cholesterol, and triglycerides may occur for which regular blood tests are needed. A physical sense of restlessness (akathisia) or agitation may occur without parents realizing that this can be a side effect. The opposite could occur as well: medication-induced parkinsonism causes decreased movement. One of the most worrisome

TABLE 16–10. Highlights of newer-generation antipsychotic adverse effects

Common

Weight gain

Muscle rigidity

Parkinsonism

Constipation

Dry mouth

Dizziness

Somnolence/fatigue

Less common

Tremors

Nausea or abdominal pain

Akathisia (restlessness)

Headache

Agitation

Orthostasis

Elevated glucose level

Elevated levels of cholesterol and triglycerides

Notable rare reactions

Tardive dyskinesia

Neuroleptic malignant syndrome

Lowered blood cell counts

Elevated liver enzymes

Prolonged QT interval

Tachycardia

but rare reactions is neuroleptic malignant syndrome, which is a severe febrile, systemic allergic reaction that may occur typically in the first few months of use (Neuhut et al. 2009). Families also must be warned about a small, but cumulative and dose-related, risk of tardive dyskinesia, which is a potentially permanent repetitive involuntary movement disorder caused by antipsychotics. Although rare, this possibility needs to be part of the ongoing risk-benefit analysis around use of these medications. Tardive dyskinesia monitoring (Table 16–11) usually involves biannual examinations with the

TABLE 16–11. Suggestions for monitoring of newer-generation antipsychotics

Record height and weight growth curve at baseline and at each follow-up, at least every 6 months.

Measure blood pressure and pulse rate at baseline and after initiation of medication.

Monitor levels of fasting blood glucose, triglycerides, and cholesterol every 6 months.

Obtain complete blood cell count with differential once after initiation.

Inform family about home monitoring for neuroleptic malignant syndrome and tardive dyskinesia.

Administer Abnormal Involuntary Movement Scale (AIMS) every 6 months.

Adjust medication until remission is achieved.

Repeat the risk-benefit analysis every 6 months to wean off the medication when appropriate.

Abnormal Involuntary Movement Scale (AIMS) for any new-onset abnormal involuntary movements (McClellan and Stock 2013).

Recording Adverse Medication Effects

If a child or an adolescent experiences an adverse effect of a medication prescribed for the treatment of a mental disorder, DSM-5 provides direction on how to record this information in the medical record (American Psychiatric Association 2013, pp. 709–714). We include Table 16–12 as a shorthand list so that you can record a movement disorder or other adverse medication effect that is a focus of clinical attention or that may otherwise affect the diagnosis, course, prognosis, or treatment of a patient's mental disorder. A condition listed in the table may be coded if it is a reason for the current visit or helps to explain the need for a test, procedure, or treatment. Conditions and problems from this list also may be included in the medical record as useful information on circumstances that may affect the patient's care, regardless of their relevance to the current visit.

TABLE 16–12. ICD-10-CM codes for adverse medication effects

ICD-10-CM code	Disorder, condition, or problem
G21.11	Neuroleptic-induced parkinsonism
G21.19	Other medication-induced parkinsonism
G21.0	Neuroleptic malignant syndrome
G24.02	Medication-induced acute dystonia
G25.71	Medication-induced acute akathisia
G24.01	Tardive dyskinesia
G24.09	Tardive dystonia
G25.71	Tardive akathisia
G25.1	Medication-induced postural tremor
G25.79	Other medication-induced movement disorder
T43.205A	Antidepressant discontinuation syndrome: initial encounter
T43.205D	Antidepressant discontinuation syndrome: subsequent encounter
T43.205S	Antidepressant discontinuation syndrome: sequelae
T50.905A	Other adverse effect of medication: initial encounter
T50.905D	Other adverse effect of medication: subsequent encounter
T50.905S	Other adverse effect of medication: sequelae

Source. World Health Organization 1992.

Chapter 17

Ideas for Practice, Education, and Research

Every day, we hear about a child or an adolescent who needs mental health care but cannot secure the care she needs. Every day, we meet an adult whose mental distress and illness went unrecognized and unaddressed in her own formative years. We know that the needs for mental health services for children and adolescents are unmet. Our guess is that any readers of this book will know that need.

As academic psychiatrists, we are grateful for our opportunities to care for patients as practitioners, to teach students and trainees to someday replace us as practitioners, and to conduct research that informs the clinical practice of other practitioners. However, we cannot accept every opportunity for clinical care, teaching, and research that is presented.

We cannot even accept the ideas that simply occur to us. Like many academics, we keep lists of ideas we hope to get to but realize that we would be fortunate to be able to address fewer than half of them. To end this book, we are offering a decidedly incomplete list of 30 ideas for practice, education, and research. We offer this incomplete conclusion both as a reminder that the work of caring for children and adolescents in mental distress is incomplete and as an invitation to join us in improving the lives of young people with mental illness. Select an idea, read the available literature on the idea, find academic or community partners to help you, and then begin.

Practice

1. Recognize and reduce adverse childhood experiences.
2. Minimize antipsychotic use, especially antipsychotic polypharmacy, among children and adolescents without psychotic disorders.

3. Develop outcome-based and quality-improvement measures that are aligned with the goals of patients and caregivers rather than with those of third-party payers and regulators.
4. Reduce the use of seclusion and restraint in pediatric psychiatric hospitals.
5. Increase the adoption rate for children in long-term foster care.
6. Use social media peer networks to deliver some forms of mental health services.
7. Increase the use of specific DSM-5 (American Psychiatric Association 2013) diagnoses, as opposed to unspecified and otherwise specified, in community settings.
8. Decrease stigma, both public and professional, about mental illness and mental health care.
9. Increase access to evidence-based behavioral- and psychological-based treatments for mental illness in children and adolescents.
10. Increase mental health service referral success rates through addressing access barriers.

Education

1. Develop community-based mental health delivery systems in nonspecialty settings.
2. Innovate curriculum for more effectively teaching mental health diagnosis and treatment to nonspecialty practitioners.
3. Teach culturally informed care that takes into account a young person's ethnicity, language, faith, and sexual orientation.
4. Develop strategies to ensure that high-quality early childhood education is available to all children.
5. Teach individual caregivers ways to maintain and strengthen the resiliency of children.
6. Incorporate mental health training into training of coaches, teachers, and other adults in caring professions.
7. Increase understanding of the effects of adverse childhood experiences and reduce their incidence.
8. Teach parents and caregivers the benefits of predictable habits at home and school for a child's development.
9. Help educators understand and implement effective strategies to prevent and reduce bullying.

10. Use public health strategies to promote greater use of effective parenting practices.

Research

1. Improve the reliability of the disruptive mood dysregulation disorder diagnosis and evaluate its best treatment in children and adolescents.
2. Study cannabis and its association with causing psychotic changes in adolescents.
3. Evaluate the childhood risk rate of tardive dyskinesia from newer-generation antipsychotics.
4. Do comparative study of interventions for child mental health conditions—for example, what is the most effective treatment for pediatric bipolar disorder?
5. Study long-term outcomes (including undesired effects) from the use of all psychotropic medications in children.
6. Test the effectiveness in children of antidepressants released over the past decade.
7. Study α_2 agonists and selective serotonin reuptake inhibitors for their degree of benefit for childhood posttraumatic stress disorder symptoms.
8. Study the potential benefits of computer-delivered (i.e., via video game, texting, and social media formats) psychosocial interventions on child mental health symptoms.
9. Study psychotherapeutic interventions (such as dialectical behavior therapy) specifically for their ability to reduce suicidality risks among high-risk adolescents.
10. Study psychosocial and behavioral interventions for autism spectrum disorders that may be more practical to implement than full-time applied behavior analysis therapy.

Integration of Care

Finally, there is a growing recognition that integrating mental and physical health services for young people will improve the experience of care and improve treatment outcomes, while (potentially) reducing the total cost of care. The jury is still out on that last point, but it has become accepted that better integration of care can make it easier for families to access services and that this integration can yield improved treatment outcomes. What remains undetermined is the particular design or way that this integration of care should work in child mental health. Over the next decade, we hope to witness and participate in major improvements in integrated care systems.

As you see children and adolescents for care, consider whether the system in which you are seeing them could be transformed into an effective integrated care system for children and adolescents. The American Academy of Child and Adolescent Psychiatry described what they thought an integrated care system should include in order to function well for both providers and families. That summary of desired elements in integrated care appears in Table 17-1.

TABLE 17–1. Elements of an effective integrated mental health care system for young people

---

1. Screening for the early detection of behavioral health problems

2. Triage or referral to appropriate behavioral health treatment

3. Ready access to child and adolescent psychiatric consultations, including:

    a. On-demand, indirect ("curbside") psychiatric consultation to the primary care provider

    b. Timely, face-to-face consultations with the patient and/or family by the child and adolescent psychiatrist

4. Care coordination that facilitates the delivery of mental health services and enhances collaboration with the health care team, parents, family, and child-serving agencies

5. Access to child psychiatric specialty treatment services for children and adolescents with moderate to severe psychiatric disorders

6. A mechanism to monitor outcomes at both the individual case and the delivery system level

---

References

Achenbach TM: Manual for the Child Behavior Checklist/4–18 and 1991 Profile. Burlington, Department of Psychiatry, University of Vermont, 1991

Achenbach TM: Manual for the Child Behavior Checklist/2–3 and 1992 Profile. Burlington, Department of Psychiatry, University of Vermont, 1992

Alarcón RD, Frank JB: The Psychotherapy of Hope: The Legacy of Persuasion and Healing. Baltimore, MD, Johns Hopkins University Press, 2011

American Academy of Child and Adolescent Psychiatry: Best Principles for Integration of Child Psychiatry Into the Pediatric Health Home, June 2012. Available at: https://www.aacap.org/App_Themes/AACAP/docs/clinical_practice_center/systems_of_care/best_principles_for_integration_of_child_psychiatry_into_the_pediatric_health_home_2012.pdf. Accessed August 31, 2015.

American Academy of Child and Adolescent Psychiatry (AACAP): Facts for Families document Web site. 2015. Available at: http://www.aacap.org/AACAP/Families_and_Youth/Facts_for_Families/Facts_for_Families_Keyword.aspx. Accessed August 31, 2015.

American Psychiatric Association: Diagnostic and Statistical Manual of Mental Disorders, 3rd Edition. Washington, DC, American Psychiatric Association, 1980

American Psychiatric Association: Diagnostic and Statistical Manual of Mental Disorders, 4th Edition. Washington, DC, American Psychiatric Association, 1994

American Psychiatric Association: Diagnostic and Statistical Manual of Mental Disorders, 4th Edition, Text Revision. Washington, DC, American Psychiatric Association, 2000

American Psychiatric Association: Diagnostic and Statistical Manual of Mental Disorders, 5th Edition. Arlington, VA, American Psychiatric Association, 2013

American Psychiatric Association: Understanding Mental Disorders: Your Guide to DSM-5. Arlington, VA, American Psychiatric Association, 2015

Bäärnhielm S, Scarpinati Rosso M: The cultural formulation: a model to combine nosology and patients' life context in psychiatric diagnostic practice. Transcult Psychiatry 46(3):406–428, 2009 19837779

Beloglovsky M, Daly L: Early Learning Theories Made Visible. St. Paul, MN, Redleaf Press, 2015

Berganza CE, Mezzich JE, Jorge MR: Latin American Guide for Psychiatric Diagnosis (GLDP). Psychopathology 35(2–3):185–190, 2002 12145508

Birmaher B, Brent D, Bernet W, et al: Practice parameter for the assessment and treatment of children and adolescents with depressive disorders. J Am Acad Child Adolesc Psychiatry 46(11):1503–1526, 2007 18049300

Birmaher B, Gill MK, Axelson DA, et al: Longitudinal trajectories and associated baseline predictors in youths with bipolar spectrum disorders. Am J Psychiatry 171(9):990–999, 2014 24874203

Bridge JA, Iyengar S, Salary CB, et al: Clinical response and risk for reported suicidal ideation and suicide attempts in pediatric antidepressant treatment: a meta-analysis of randomized controlled trials. JAMA 297(15):1683–1696, 2007 17440145

Buu A, Dipiazza C, Wang J, et al: Parent, family, and neighborhood effects on the development of child substance use and other psychopathology from preschool to the start of adulthood. J Stud Alcohol Drugs 70(4):489–498, 2009 19515288

Buxton D, Potter MP, Bostic JQ: Coping strategies for child bully-victims. Pediatr Ann 42(4):57–61, 2013 23556519

Cepeda C: Clinical Manual for the Psychiatric Interview of Children and Adolescents. Arlington, VA, American Psychiatric Association, 2010

Chen YF: Chinese Classification of Mental Disorders (CCMD-3): towards integration in international classification. Psychopathology 35(2–3):171–175, 2002 12145505

Chorpita BF, Daleiden EL: Mapping evidence-based treatments for children and adolescents: application of the distillation and matching model to 615 treatments from 322 randomized trials. J Consult Clin Psychol 77(3):566–579, 2009 19485596

Christophersen ER, VanScoyoc SW: Treatments That Work With Children: Empirically Supported Strategies for Managing Childhood Problems, 2nd Edition. Washington, DC, American Psychological Association, 2013

Cohen H: The nature, methods and purpose of diagnosis. Lancet 24(6227):23–25, 1943

Correll CU, Manu P, Olshanskiy V, et al: Cardiometabolic risk of second-generation antipsychotic medications during first-time use in children and adolescents. JAMA 302(16):1765–1773, 2009 19861668

Davanzo R, Copertino M, De Cunto A, et al: Antidepressant drugs and breastfeeding: a review of the literature. Breastfeed Med 6(2):89–98, 2011 20958101

de Haan AM, Boon AE, de Jong JT, et al: A meta-analytic review on treatment dropout in child and adolescent outpatient mental health care. Clin Psychol Rev 33(5):698–711, 2013 23742782

Digman JM: Personality structure: emergence of the five-factor model. Annu Rev Psychol 41:417–440, 1990

Dvir Y, Ford JD, Hill M, Frazier JA: Childhood maltreatment, emotional dysregulation, and psychiatric comorbidities. Harv Rev Psychiatry 22(3):149–161, 2014 24704784

Eaton DK, Kann L, Kinchen S, et al; Centers for Disease Control and Prevention (CDC): Youth risk behavior surveillance— United States, 2007. MMWR Surveill Summ 57(4):1–131, 2008 18528314

Egger HL, Emde RN: Developmentally sensitive diagnostic criteria for mental health disorders in early childhood: the Diagnostic and Statistical Manual of Mental Disorders-IV, the Research Diagnostic Criteria-Preschool Age, and the Diagnostic Classification of Mental Health and Developmental Disorders of Infancy and Early Childhood-Revised. Am Psychol 66(2):95–106, 2011 21142337

Emanuel EJ, Emanuel LL: Four models of the physician-patient relationship. JAMA 267(16):2221–2226, 1992 1556799

Emslie GJ, Mayes T, Porta G, et al: Treatment of Resistant Depression in Adolescents (TORDIA): week 24 outcomes. Am J Psychiatry 167(7):782–791, 2010 20478877

Estroff SE, Henderson GE: Social and cultural contributions to health, difference, and inequality, in The Social Medicine Reader, 2nd Edition, Vol 2. Edited by Henderson G, Estroff, SE. Durham, NC, Duke University Press, 2005, pp 4–26

Fairburn CG, Bohn K: Eating disorder NOS (EDNOS): an example of the troublesome "not otherwise specified" (NOS) category in DSM-IV. Behav Res Ther 43(6):691–701, 2005 15890163

Feinstein AR: Clinical Judgment. Baltimore, MD, Williams & Wilkins, 1967

First MB: DSM-5 Handbook of Differential Diagnosis. Washington, DC, American Psychiatric Publishing, 2014

Folstein MF, Folstein SE, McHugh PR: "Mini-mental state": a practical method for grading the cognitive state of patients for the clinician. J Psychiatr Res 12(3):189–198, 1975 1202204

Ford CA, Millstein SG, Halpern-Felsher BL, Irwin CE Jr: Influence of physician confidentiality assurances on adolescents' willingness to disclose information and seek future health care: a randomized controlled trial. JAMA 278(12):1029–1034, 1997 9307357

Gerber RJ, Wilks T, Erdie-Lalena C: Developmental milestones: motor development. Pediatr Rev 31(7):267–276, quiz 277, 2010a 20595440

Gerber RJ, Wilks T, Erdie-Lalena C: Developmental milestones: cognitive development. Pediatr Rev 31(9):364–367, 2010b 20810700

Gerber RJ, Wilks T, Erdie-Lalena C: Developmental milestones 3: social-emotional development. Pediatr Rev 32(12):533–536, 2011 22135423

Gold MA, Seningen AE: Interviewing adolescents, in American Academy of Pediatrics Textbook of Pediatric Care. Edited by McInerny TK. Washington, DC, American Academy of Pediatrics, 2009, pp 1331–1337

Hanington L, Ramchandani P, Stein A: Parental depression and child temperament: assessing child to parent effects in a longitudinal population study. Infant Behav Dev 33(1):88–95, 2010 20056283

Hanley GP, Iwata BA, McCord BE: Functional analysis of problem behavior: a review. J Appl Behav Anal 36(2):147–185, 2003 12858983

Hazell P, Mirzaie M: Tricyclic drugs for depression in children and adolescents. Cochrane Database Syst Rev 6:CD002317, 2013 23780719

Hilt RJ: Monitoring psychiatric medications in children. Pediatr Ann 41(4):157–163, 2012 22494208

Hilt RJ: Primary Care Principles for Child Mental Health, Version 5.0. 2014. Available at: www.palforkids.org/resources.html. Accessed August 31, 2015.

Insel T, Cuthbert B, Garvey M, et al: Research Domain Criteria (RDoC): toward a new classification framework for research on mental disorders. Am J Psychiatry 167(7):748–751, 2010 20595427

Jellinek M, Patel BP, Froehle MC (eds): Bright Futures in Practice: Mental Health, Vol. 1: Practice Guide. Arlington, VA, National Center for Education in Maternal and Child Health, 2002. Available at: www.brightfutures.org/mentalhealth. Accessed August 31, 2015.

Jonas BS, Gu Q, Albertorio-Diaz JR: Psychotropic Medication Use Among Adolescents: United States, 2005–2010 (NCHS Data Brief, No 135). Hyattsville, MD, National Center for Health Statistics, 2013

Kendall PC: Child and Adolescent Therapy: Cognitive-Behavioral Procedures, 4th Edition. New York, Guilford, 2012

Kendell R, Jablensky A: Distinguishing between the validity and utility of psychiatric diagnoses. Am J Psychiatry 160(1):4–12, 2003 12505793

Kendler KS: The dappled nature of causes of psychiatric illness: replacing the organic-functional/hardware-software dichotomy with empirically based pluralism. Mol Psychiatry 17(4):377–388, 2012 22230881

Kessler RC, Chiu WT, Demler O, et al: Prevalence, severity, and comorbidity of 12-month DSM-IV disorders in the National Comorbidity Survey Replication [published erratum appears in Arch Gen Psychiatry 62:709, 200]. Arch Gen Psychiatry 62(6):617–627, 2005 15939839

Kinghorn WA: Whose disorder?: a constructive MacIntyrean critique of psychiatric nosology. J Med Philos 36(2):187–205, 2011 21357652

Knight JR, Sherritt L, Shrier LA, et al: Validity of the CRAFFT substance abuse screening test among adolescent clinic patients. Arch Pediatr Adolesc Med 156(6):607–614, 2002 12038895

Lanza di Scalea T, Wisner KL: Antidepressant medication use during breastfeeding. Clin Obstet Gynecol 52(3):483–497, 2009 19661763

Lavigne JV, Lebailly SA, Gouze KR, et al: Treating oppositional defiant disorder in primary care: a comparison of three models. J Pediatr Psychol 33(5):449–461, 2008 17956932

Lewis SP, Heath NL: Nonsuicidal self-injury among youth. J Pediatr 166(3):526–530, 2015 25596101

Lewis-Fernández R, Aggarwal NK, Hinton L, et al: DSM-5 Handbook on the Cultural Formulation Interview. Arlington, VA, American Psychiatric Association, 2015

Lieberman J: Shrinks: The Untold Story of Psychiatry. New York, Little, Brown, 2015

Lim R: Clinical Manual of Cultural Psychiatry, 2nd Edition. Arlington, VA, American Psychiatric Association, 2015

Lizardi D, Oquendo MA, Graver R: Clinical pitfalls in the diagnosis of ataque de nervios: a case study. Transcult Psychiatry 46(3):463–486, 2009 19837782

Loy JH, Merry SN, Hetrick SE, Stasiak K: Atypical antipsychotics for disruptive behaviour disorders in children and youths. Cochrane Database Syst Rev 6:CD008559, 2012 22972123

MacIntyre AC: Dependent Rational Animals: Why Human Beings Need the Virtues. Chicago, IL, Open Court Publishing, 2012

Martínez LC: DSM-IV-TR cultural formulation of psychiatric cases: two proposals for clinicians. Transcult Psychiatry 46(3):506–523, 2009 19837784

Mash EJ, Barkley RA: Assessment of Childhood Disorders, 4th Edition. New York, Guilford, 2007

McCartney K, Philips DA: Blackwell Handbook of Early Childhood Development. Malden, MA, Blackwell, 2006

McClellan J, Stock S; American Academy of Child and Adolescent Psychiatry (AACAP) Committee on Quality Issues (CQI): Practice parameter for the assessment and treatment of children and adolescents with schizophrenia. J Am Acad Child Adolesc Psychiatry 52(9):976–990, 2013 23972700

McLaughlin MR: Speech and language delay in children. Am Fam Physician 83(10):1183–1188, 2011 21568252

McVoy M, Findling RL: Clinical Manual of Child and Adolescent Psychopharmacology, 2nd Edition. Washington, DC, American Psychiatric Publishing, 2013

Meltzer LJ, Johnson C, Crosette J, et al: Prevalence of diagnosed sleep disorders in pediatric primary care practices. Pediatrics 125(6):e1410–e1418, 2010 20457689

Merikangas KR, He JP, Burstein M, et al: Lifetime prevalence of mental disorders in U.S. adolescents: results from the National Comorbidity Survey Replication—Adolescent Supplement (NCS-A). J Am Acad Child Adolesc Psychiatry 49(10):980–989, 2010 20855043

Mindell J, Owens J: A Clinical Guide to Pediatric Sleep: Diagnosis and Management of Pediatric Sleep Problems, 2nd Edition. Philadelphia, PA, Lippincott, Williams & Wilkins, 2009

Mises R, Quemada N, Botbol M, et al: French classification for child and adolescent mental disorders. Psychopathology 35(2–3):176–180, 2002 12145506

Mohatt J, Bennett SM, Walkup JT: Treatment of separation, generalized, and social anxiety disorders in youths. Am J Psychiatry 171(7):741–748, 2014 24874020

Mooney CG: Theories of Childhood: An Introduction to Dewey, Montessori, Erikson, Piaget, and Vygotsky, 2nd Edition. St. Paul, MN, Redleaf Press, 2013

Murthy S, Mandl KD, Bourgeois F: Analysis of pediatric clinical drug trials for neuropsychiatric conditions. Pediatrics 131(6):1125–1131, 2013 23650305

Nakane Y, Nakane H: Classification systems for psychiatric diseases currently used in Japan. Psychopathology 35(2–3):191–194, 2002 12145509

Neuhut R, Lindenmayer J-P, Silva R: Neuroleptic malignant syndrome in children and adolescents on atypical antipsychotic medication: a review. J Child Adolesc Psychopharmacol 19(4):415–422, 2009 19702493

Nurcombe B: Diagnosis and treatment planning in child and adolescent mental health problems, in IACAPAP e-Textbook of Child and Adolescent Mental Health. Edited by Rey JM. Geneva, Switzerland, International Association for Child and Adolescent Psychiatry and Allied Professions, 2014, pp 1–21.

Nussbaum AM: Pocket Guide to the DSM-5 Diagnostic Exam. Washington, DC, American Psychiatric Publishing, 2013

Otero-Ojeda AA: Third Cuban Glossary of Psychiatry (GC-3): key features and contributions. Psychopathology 35(2–3):181–184, 2002 12145507

Paschetta E, Berrisford G, Coccia F, et al: Perinatal psychiatric disorders: an overview. Am J Obstet Gynecol 210(6):501–509.e6, 2014 24113256

Pearlstein T: Use of psychotropic medication during pregnancy and the postpartum period. Womens Health (Lond Engl) 9(6):605–615, 2013 24161312

Phillips J, Frances A, Cerullo MA, et al: The six most essential questions in psychiatric diagnosis: a pluralogue part 1: conceptual and definitional issues in psychiatric diagnosis. Philos Ethics Humanit Med 7:3, 2012a 22243994

Phillips J, Frances A, Cerullo MA, et al: The six most essential questions in psychiatric diagnosis: a pluralogue part 2: issues of conservatism and pragmatism in psychiatric diagnosis. Philos Ethics Humanit Med 7:8, 2012b 22512887

Phillips J, Frances A, Cerullo MA, et al: The six most essential questions in psychiatric diagnosis: a pluralogue part 3: issues of utility and alternative approaches in psychiatric diagnosis. Philos Ethics Humanit Med 7:9, 2012c 22621419

Preston J, O'Neal JH, Talaga MC: Child and Adolescent Clinical Psychopharmacology Made Simple, 3rd Edition. Oakland, CA, New Harbinger Publications, 2015

Pringsheim T, Steeves T: Pharmacological treatment for attention deficit hyperactivity disorder (ADHD) in children with comorbid tic disorders. Cochrane Database Syst Rev (4):CD007990, 2011 21491404

Radden J, Sadler JZ: The Virtuous Psychiatrist: Character Ethics in Psychiatric Practice. New York, Oxford University Press, 2010

Reynolds CR, Kamphaus RW: BASC: Behavior Assessment System for Children: Manual. Circle Pines, MN, American Guidance Service, 1998

Romano E, Babchishin L, Marquis R, Fréchette S: Childhood maltreatment and educational outcomes. Trauma Violence Abuse 16(4):418–437, 2015 24920354

Roos J, Werbart A: Therapist and relationship factors influencing dropout from individual psychotherapy: a literature review. Psychother Res 23(4):394–418, 2013 23461273

Roy AK, Lopes V, Klein RG: Disruptive mood dysregulation disorder: a new diagnostic approach to chronic irritability in youth. Am J Psychiatry 171(9):918–924, 2014 25178749

Rushton J, Bruckman D, Kelleher K: Primary care referral of children with psychosocial problems. Arch Pediatr Adolesc Med 156(6):592–598, 2002 12038893

Safer DJ, Rajakannan T, Burcu M, Zito JM: Trends in subthreshold psychiatric diagnoses for youth in community treatment. JAMA Psychiatry 72(1):75–83, 2015 25426673

Satyanarayana VA, Lukose A, Srinivasan K: Maternal mental health in pregnancy and child behavior. Indian J Psychiatry 53(4):351–361, 2011 22303046

Scott BG, Sanders AFP, Graham RA, et al: Identity distress among youth exposed to natural disasters: associations with level of exposure, posttraumatic stress, and internalizing problems. Identity (Mahwah, N J) 14(4):255–267, 2014 25505851

Shahrokh NC, Hales RE, Phillips KA, et al: The Language of Mental Health: A Glossary of Psychiatric Terms. Washington, DC, American Psychiatric Publishing, 2011

Silber TJ: Somatization disorders: diagnosis, treatment, and prognosis. Pediatr Rev 32(2):56–63, quiz 63–64, 2011 21285301

Stubbe D: Child and Adolescent Psychiatry: A Practical Guide. Philadelphia, PA, Lippincott Williams & Wilkins, 2007

Substance Abuse and Mental Health Services Administration: Results From the 2013 National Survey on Drug Use and Health: Summary of National Findings (NSDUH Series H-48, HHS Publ No SMA 14-4863). Rockville, MD, Substance Abuse and Mental Health Services Administration, 2014

Summers RF, Barber JP: Therapeutic alliance as a measurable psychotherapy skill. Acad Psychiatry 27(3):160–165, 2003 12969839

Task Force on Research Diagnostic Criteria: Infancy Preschool: Research diagnostic criteria for infants and preschool children: the process and empirical support. J Am Acad Child Adolesc Psychiatry 42(12):1504–1512, 2003 14627886

Trivedi HK, Kershner JD: Practical Child and Adolescent Psychiatry for Pediatrics and Primary Care. Cambridge, MA, Hogrefe, 2009

U.S. Food and Drug Administration: Online label repository, 1999. Available at http://labels.fda.gov. Accessed March 1, 2015.

U.S. Public Health Service Office of the Surgeon General: Mental Health: A Report of the Surgeon General. Rockville, MD, U.S. Department of Health and Human Services, U.S. Public Health Service, 1999

van Nierop M, Janssens M; Genetic Risk Outcome of Psychosis Investigators, et al: Evidence that transition from health to psychotic disorder can be traced to semi-ubiquitous environmental effects operating against background genetic risk. PLoS One 8(11):e76690, 2013 24223116

Vernon-Feagans L, Garrett-Peters P, Willoughby M, Mills-Koonce R; The Family Life Project Key Investigators: Chaos, poverty, and parenting: predictors of early language development. Early Child Res Q 27(3):339–351, 2012 23049162

Weisz JR, Kazdin AE: Evidence-Based Psychotherapies for Children and Adolescents, 2nd Edition. New York, Guilford, 2010

World Health Organization: International Classification of Diseases, 9th Revision, Clinical Modification. Ann Arbor, MI, Commission on Professional and Hospital Activities, 1978

World Health Organization: The ICD-10 Classification of Mental and Behavioural Disorders: Clinical Descriptions and Diagnostic Guidelines. Geneva, World Health Organization, 1992

Yuma-Guerrero PJ, Lawson KA, Velasquez MM, et al: Screening, brief intervention, and referral for alcohol use in adolescents: a systematic review. Pediatrics 130(1):115–122, 2012 22665407

Zero to Three: Diagnostic Classification of Mental Health and Developmental Disorders of Infancy and Early Childhood (DC:0–3). Arlington, VA, Zero to Three/National Center for Clinical Infant Programs, 1994

Zero to Three: Diagnostic Classification of Mental Health and Developmental Disorders of Infancy and Early Childhood, Revised (DC:0–3R). Washington, DC, Zero to Three, 2005

Index

Page numbers printed in **boldface** type refer to tables or figures.

Ability, and academic
    performance, 22, 24
Abnormal Involuntary
    Movement Scale
    (AIMS), 298
Abuse, childhood
    anxious or avoidant
        behavior and, **38**
    caregivers and, 191
    developmental delay and,
        26
    disruptive or aggressive
        behavior and, **30**
    Early Development and
        Home Background
        form and, 214
    15-minute pediatric
        diagnostic interview
        and, 63
    irritable or labile mood
        and, **36**
    poor academic performance
        and, **23**, 24
    recurrent and excessive
        physical complaints
        and, **42**
    sleep problems and, **45**
    withdrawn or sad mood
        and, **33**
Acute stress disorder, 116
Adaptive skills
    developmental milestones
        and, 242–243, **244–245**

intellectual disability and
    deficits in, 86, 243
ADHD. *See* Attention-deficit/
    hyperactivity disorder
ADHD Rating Scale-IV, **230**
Adjustment disorder
    posttraumatic stress
        disorder and, 116
    psychosocial stressors and,
        193
    recurrent and excessive
        physical complaints
        and, **42**
    withdrawn or sad mood
        and, 32, **33**
Adolescents. *See also* Age
    age-based behavioral
        screening of, 17, **18–19**
    Cultural Formulation
        Interview and, 213–214
    gender dysphoria in, 136–
        137
    prevalence of DSM-IV
        disorders in, **20**
    prevalence of self-harm and
        suicidality in, 46, 48
    prevalence of substance
        abuse in, 49
    therapeutic alliance and
        initial interviews with,
        6
    withdrawn or sad mood
        in, 32

Adverse childhood experiences, 214, 221. *See also* Abuse; Neglect; Trauma

Affect. *See* Positive emotion

Age. *See also* Adolescents; Age at onset; Infants; Preschool children; School-age children; Toddlers

behavioral health screening and, 17

for common mental disorder presentations, 16–17, **18–19**

Cultural Formulation Interview and, 213

developmental milestones and, 190, **244–247**

Ages & Stages Questionnaires (ASQ), 22

Aggression. *See also* Violence

antipsychotics for, 31, 277

cannabis withdrawal and, 151

as common clinical concern, 28–31

intermittent explosive disorder and, 139

Agoraphobia, **20**, 107

Alcohol. *See* Neurobehavioral disorder associated with prenatal alcohol exposure; Substance abuse

Alcohol intoxication, 146

Alcohol use disorder, 144–146

Alcohol withdrawal, 146

Alexithymia, 41

Allergies, and 30-minute pediatric diagnostic interview, 78

Alpha-agonists, 46

Alternative diagnoses. *See also* Differential diagnosis; *specific disorders*

use of term in context of DSM-5 pediatric diagnostic interview, 84

American Academy of Child and Adolescent Psychiatry (AACAP), 255, 276, 304

Amphetamine salt combination (Adderall), **280, 283**

Anemia, and withdrawn or sad mood, 32, **33**

Anger

cannabis withdrawal and, 151

disruptive mood dysregulation disorder and, 105

Level 1 Cross-Cutting Symptom Measure and, **210**

oppositional defiant disorder and, 138

tobacco withdrawal and, 169

Animal cruelty, and conduct disorder, 140

Anorexia nervosa

abbreviated DSM-5 criteria for, **183**

as common clinical concern, 54, **55**

DSM-5 pediatric diagnostic interview and, 124–125

modifiers for, 124–125

shorthand description of, **65**

Antagonism, and personality disorders, 222

Antihistamines, 46
Antipsychotics
    aggression and, 31, 277
    insomnia and, 46
    monitoring of, **298**
    side effects of, 296–297
Anxiety. *See also* Anxiety
        disorder(s)
    alcohol withdrawal and, 147
    cannabis withdrawal and,
        151
    as common clinical
        concern, 37–40
    illness anxiety disorder
        and, 123
    Level 1 Cross-Cutting
        Symptom Measure
        and, **211**
    rating scales for, **229**
    sedative, hypnotic, or
        anxiolytic withdrawal
        and, 163
    somatic symptom disorder
        and, 121
    30-minute pediatric
        diagnostic interview
        and questions on, 77
    tobacco withdrawal and,
        169
Anxiety disorder(s). *See also*
        Anxiety
    abbreviated DSM-5 criteria
        for, **179**
    age of onset for, 16
    cognitive-behavioral
        therapy for, **270**
    DSM-5 pediatric diagnostic
        interview and, 106–110
    group therapy for, **271**
    medications for, **287–289**
    poor academic
        performance and, **23**

postpartum maternal
        mental health and, **57**
    recurrent and excessive
        physical complaints
        and, **42**
    relaxation training for, **273**
    self-harm or suicidality
        and, 49
Appearance, and mental
        status examination, 195
Appetite
    cannabis intoxication and
        increased, 150
    cannabis withdrawal and
        decreased, 151
    stimulant withdrawal and
        increased, 167
    tobacco withdrawal and
        increased, 169
Applied behavioral analysis,
        272
Argumentative behavior, and
        oppositional defiant
        disorder, 138
Aripiprazole, **290,** 296
Atomoxetine, **285**
Attention, opioid intoxication
        and impairment of, 159.
        See also Concentration;
        Distractibility; Inattention
Attention-deficit/
        hyperactivity disorder
        (ADHD)
    abbreviated DSM-5 criteria
        for, **176**
    alternative diagnoses for, 94
    disruptive or aggressive
        behavior and, 29, **30**
    DSM-5 pediatric diagnostic
        interview and, 91–94
    medications and treatment
        of, 268, **278–286, 294**

Attention-deficit/
hyperactivity disorder
(ADHD) *(continued)*
modifiers for, 93
poor academic performance
and, **23**, 25
prevalence of, **20**
rating scales for, **230**
shorthand description of,
65
social skills training for, **273**
Atypical presentations, and
symptoms related to
medical conditions, 192
Autism spectrum disorder
abbreviated DSM-5 criteria
for, **176**
alternative diagnoses for,
90–91
applied behavioral
analysis for, **272**
developmental delay and,
26
disruptive behavior and, 29
DSM-5 pediatric diagnostic
interview and, 88–91
modifiers for, 90
rating scales for, **231**
shorthand description of, **65**
social-emotional
development and, 27
social skills training for, **273**
Autism-Spectrum Quotient
(AQ), **231**
Avoidant behavior
as common clinical
concern, 37–40
specific phobia and, 106
Avoidant/restrictive food
intake disorder, 125–126

Behavior. *See also* Aggression;
Anger; Anxiety; Avoidant
behavior; Disruptive
behavior; Risky behaviors
autism spectrum disorder
and routines of, 89
functional analysis of, 28–
29, 259–260
mental status examination
and, 195
rating scales and, **229**
Behavioral activation, 260–261
Behavior Assessment System
for Children, 61
Behavior management
training, 31, 37, 268, **272**
Benzodiazepines, 45, 46
Best practices, and treatment
goals, 255
Beta-blockers, 32
Bibliotherapy, 13
Bipolar disorder
abbreviated DSM-5 criteria
for, **178**
alternative diagnoses for,
99, 101
DSM-5 pediatric diagnostic
interview and, 97–101
disruptive mood
dysregulation
disorder and, 106
irritable or labile mood
and, 35, **36**
medications for, **290–292**
modifiers for, 98–99, 100–
101
prevalence of, **20**
self-harm or suicidality
and, **47**
shorthand description of, **65**

withdrawn or sad mood and, **33,** 34

Blood pressure, and stimulant intoxication, 166

Body dysmorphic disorder, 112

Body-focused repetitive behaviors, 113

Body image, and anorexia nervosa, 124

Bradycardia, and stimulant intoxication, 166

Breath and breathing, and panic disorder, 108

Brief assessment, and diagnosis in community setting, 11

Brief Dissociative Experiences Scale (DES-B), **233**

Brief Impairment Scale, **229**

Brief psychotic disorder, 96

Bulimia nervosa, **55, 65,** 125, **183**

Bullying
anxious or avoidant behavior and, **38**
conduct disorder and, 140
developmental delay and, **26**
disruptive or aggressive behavior and, **30**
poor academic performance and, **23,** 24
psychosocial interventions and, 261–263
sleep problems and, **45**
withdrawn or sad mood and, **33**

Caffeine intoxication, 147–148

Caffeine withdrawal, 148–149

Cannabis intoxication, 150–151

Cannabis use disorder, 149–150

Cannabis withdrawal, 151–152

Cardiac arrhythmia, and caffeine intoxication, 148

Caregivers. *See also* Family; Parents
coaching of on appropriate use of psychotherapy, 14
Cultural Formulation Interview and, 214
Early Development and Home Background form and, 221
oppositional defiant disorder and mismatch in, 29
postcrisis planning for, 263–265
reactive attachment disorder and repeated changes of, 117
self-help strategies for in community settings, 13
symptoms related to conflict with, 190–191
treatment plans and goals of, 253–255

Cataplexy, and narcolepsy, 131, 132

Catatonia, 95

Categorical model, of mental illness, 199

CBT. *See* Cognitive-behavioral therapy

Cell phones, and insomnia, 43–44

Center for Epidemiologic
    Studies Depression Scale
    for Children (CES-DC),
    230
Central sleep apnea, 133
CFI. *See* Cultural
    Formulation Interview
Chest pains, and panic
    disorder, 108
Child Behavior Checklist, 61
Child-directed play, and
    special time, 258
Childhood Autism Spectrum
    Test (CAST), **231**
Childhood-onset fluency
    disorder, 88
Children. *See* Abuse;
    Adolescents; Adverse
    childhood experiences;
    Age; Infants; Neglect;
    Patients; Preschool
    children; School-age
    children; Toddlers
Children's Revised Impact of
    Events Scale-8 (CRIES-
    8), **230**
Chills
    panic disorder and, 108
    stimulant intoxication
        and, 166
Chlorpromazine, 277
Choking, panic disorder and
    fear of, 108
Circadian rhythm sleep-wake
    disorder, 129
Citalopram, 35, **287**
Clinical concerns, common
    anxious or avoidant
        behavior as, 37–40
    development delay as, 25–
        28
    disruptive or aggressive
        behavior as, 28–31

disturbed eating as, 54
irritable or labile mood as,
    35–37
poor academic
    performance as, 22–25
postpartum maternal
    mental health as, 54–57
recurrent and excessive
    physical complaints
    as, 40–43
self-harm and suicidality
    as, 46–49
sleep problems as, 43–46
substance abuse as, 49–54
withdrawn or sad mood
    as, 32–35
Clinician-Rated Dimensions
    of Psychosis Symptom
    Severity, **233**
Clinician-Rated Severity of
    Autism Spectrum and
    Social Communication
    Disorders, **233**
Clinician-Rated Severity of
    Conduct Disorder, **233**
Clinician-Rated Severity of
    Nonsuicidal Self-Injury,
    233
Clinician-Rated Severity of
    Oppositional Defiant
    Disorder, **233**
Clinician-Rated Severity of
    Somatic Symptom
    Disorder, **233**
Clomipramine, **289**
Clonidine, 31, **285, 286**
Codes and coding. *See* ICD-10
Cognition, and mental status
    examination, 197. *See
    also* Cognitive
    development; Thought

Cognitive-behavioral therapy (CBT). *See also* Trauma-focused cognitive-behavioral therapy
anxious or avoidant behavior and, 40
description of and typical indications for, **270**
Cognitive development, and developmental delays, 27, **246–247.** *See also* Cognition
Collateral information, and 30-minute pediatric diagnostic interview, 72
Columbia Impairment Scale, **229**
Coma
inhalant intoxication and, 156
opioid intoxication and, 159
Comfort seeking, and reactive attachment disorder, 117
Communication disorder. *See also* Language disorder; Speech
developmental delay and, **26**
disruptive or aggressive behavior and, **30**
intellectual disability and, 88
Community behavioral health systems. *See also* Treatment
age-based behavioral health screening in, 17
appropriate prescription of medications by, 14–15
common ages for presentations of mental disorders in, 16–17, **18–19**

diagnosis of specific mental disorders in, 11–12
education about mental health treatment and, 12–13
improvement of support for specialist services, 9
initiation of counseling and psychotherapy, 14
recognition of mental distress and, 10
screening for mental distress in, 10–11
self-help strategies for patients and caregivers, 13
Comorbidity, differential diagnosis and symptoms related to, 192–193
Compulsions
mental status examination and, 196
obsessive-compulsive disorder and, 111
30-minute pediatric diagnostic interview and, 77
Concentration. *See also* Attention; Distractibility
caffeine withdrawal and, 148
generalized anxiety disorder and, 110
posttraumatic stress disorder and, 116
tobacco withdrawal and, 169
Conduct disorder
abbreviated DSM-5 criteria for, **185**
alternative diagnoses for, 142–143

Conduct disorder (*continued*)
  behavior management
    training for, 31, **272**
  disruptive or aggressive
    behavior and, **30,** 31
  DSM-5 pediatric
    diagnostic interview
    and, 140–143
  family therapy for, **271**
  modifiers for, 141–142
  poor academic performance
    and, **23**
  prevalence of, **20**
  shorthand description of, **65**
Confidentiality
  substance abuse and, 50–51
  30-minute pediatric
    diagnostic interview
    and, 74–75
Confusion, and stimulant
  intoxication, 166
Continuous positive airway
  pressure (CPAP)
  systems, 45
Control, panic disorder and
  fear of loss of, 109
Conversation starters, for
  initial interviews, 7
Conversion disorder
  recurrent and excessive
    physical complaints
    and, **42,** 43
  somatic symptom disorder
    and, 121–122
Counseling
  initiation of in community
    settings, 14
  for irritable or labile mood,
    37
CRAFFT Screening Interview,
  51, **52–53,** 164, **230**

Cravings, and substance-
  related and addictive
  disorders, 144, 149, 152,
  155, 157, 160, 167, 170
Crisis prevention plan, 264
Cross-dressing, and gender
  dysphoria, 136
Cruelty, and conduct disorder,
  140
Cultural Formulation
  Interview (CFI), 201,
  212–214
Culture. *See also* Cultural
  Formulation Interview
  conflicts with caregivers
    and, 191
  cultural syndromes, idiom
    of distress, and
    explanations of
    perceived cause, 212
  culture-specific diagnostic
    systems and, 235
Curfews, and conduct
  disorder, 141
Cyclothymic disorder, 101

Daytime sleepiness, and
  obstructive sleep apnea,
  133
Death
  panic disorder and fear of,
    109
  suicide and leading causes
    of, 48
Defiant behavior, and
  oppositional defiant
  disorder, 138
Delusion(s)
  mental status examination
    and, 197
  schizophrenia and, 94
Delusional disorder, 96, 97

Depersonalization, and panic disorder, 108–109
Depersonalization/ derealization disorder, 119–120
Depression, and depressive disorders. *See also* Major depressive disorder; Mood disorders
abbreviated DSM-5 criteria for, **178–179**
cognitive-behavioral therapy for, **270**
DSM-5 pediatric diagnostic interview and, 101–106
family therapy for, **271**
Level 1 Cross-Cutting Symptom Measure and, **210**
medications for, **287–289**
rating scales for, **230**
recurrent and excessive physical complaints and, **42**
relaxation training for, **273**
withdrawn or sad mood and, 34
Derealization, and panic disorder, 108–109. *See also* Depersonalization/ derealization disorder
Detachment
personality disorders and, 222
posttraumatic stress disorder and, 115
Developmental coordination disorder, 90
Developmental delays. *See also* Developmental history
as common clinical concern, 25–28

influence of on age and appearance of mental disorders, 16
poor academic performance and, 22
Developmental history. *See also* Developmental delays
identification of milestones in, 241–243, **244–245**
red flags as triggers for specialized assessments of, **246–247**
symptoms related to conflict or stage of, 190
30-minute pediatric diagnostic interview and, 78
Deviation, and developmental milestones, 243
Dexmethylphenidate, **279, 282**
Dextroamphetamine, **279, 284**
Diagnosis. *See also* Alternative diagnoses
abbreviated criteria for common in DSM-5, **176–185**
in community behavioral health systems, 11–12
culture-specific systems of, 235
of neurobehavioral disorder associated with prenatal alcohol exposure, 28
problem lists and, 249–252
systems of for infants and toddlers, 235
therapeutic alliance as first step in successful, 5–6
Diagnostic Classification of Mental Health and Developmental Disorders of Infancy and Early Childhood (DC:0–3), 235

Dialectical behavior therapy, **271**

Diarrhea, and opioid withdrawal, 160

Differential diagnosis, description of stepwise approach to, 189–193. *See also* Alternative diagnoses; Diagnosis

Dimensional model, of personality disorders, 222–223

Diphenhydramine, 296

Disinhibited social engagement disorder, 118

Disorders, use of term, 251

Disorganization, and attention-deficit/ hyperactivity disorder, 92

Disproportionate reaction, and disruptive mood dysregulation disorder, 105

Disruptive behavior, as common clinical concern, 28–31

Disruptive, impulse-control, and conduct disorders abbreviated DSM-5 criteria for, **184–185**
DSM-5 pediatric diagnostic interview and, 137–138

Disruptive mood dysregulation disorder, 35, **36**, 37, 105–106, **178**

Dissociation. *See also* Dissociative disorders developmental milestones and, 243
30-minute pediatric diagnostic interview and, 77

Dissociative amnesia, 119

Dissociative disorders, 118–120. *See also* Dissociation

Dissociative identity disorder, 119

Distractibility. *See also* Attention; Concentration attention-deficit/ hyperactivity disorder and, 92
bipolar disorder and, 98, 100
mental status examination and, 196

Diuresis, and caffeine intoxication, 147

Dizziness inhalant intoxication and, 156
panic disorder and, 108

Dreams. *See also* Nightmare disorder posttraumatic stress disorder and, 114
stimulant withdrawal and, 167

Drowsiness, and opioid intoxication, 159

Dry mouth, and cannabis intoxication, 151

DSM-5. *See also* Cultural Formulation Interview; Diagnosis; DSM-5 pediatric diagnostic interview; Early Development and Home Background form; Level 1 and Level 2 Cross-Cutting Symptom Measures; Personality Inventory for DSM-5—Brief Form— Child Age 11–17

abbreviated criteria for common diagnoses in, **176–185**

categorical model of mental illness in, 199

definition of mental disorder in, 64, 227

dimensional model of personality disorders and, 222–223

requirements for well-supported diagnosis and, 11

shorthand descriptions of common diagnoses in, **65**

DSM-5 pediatric diagnostic interview. *See also specific disorders*

exclusion criteria in context of, 84

follow-up questions and, 83–84

function of alternatives in, 84

ICD-10 codes and, 85

use of suggested screening questions in, 83

Duloxetine, **289**

Dysphoria, 32

Dysthymia. *See* Persistent depressive disorder (dysthymia)

Early Childhood Screening Assessment (ECSA), **229**

Early Development and Home Background (EDHB) form, 214, **215–220**, 221

Early intervention services, referral to, 68

Eating disorders. *See also* Anorexia nervosa; Bulimia nervosa; Eating and feeding

abbreviated DSM-5 criteria for, **183**

alternative diagnoses for, 125, 126

cognitive-behavioral therapy for, **270**

DSM-5 pediatric diagnostic interview and, 123–126

family therapy for, **271**

prevalence of, **20**

Eating and feeding. *See also* Appetite; Eating disorders; Weight gain or loss

disturbed as common clinical concern, 54, **55**

30-minute pediatric diagnostic interview and, 77

Edinburgh Postnatal Depression Scale (EPDS), **231**

Education. *See also* Schools

on mental health treatment in community settings, 12–13

bullying and, 262

recommendations for, 302–303

substance use disorder and, 54

Elimination, and 30-minute pediatric diagnostic interview, 77

Elimination disorders

abbreviated DSM-5 criteria for, **183**

Elimination disorders
(continued)
DSM-5 pediatric diagnostic
interview and, 126–128
modifiers for, 127, 1258
Emergency departments
postcrisis planning for
caregivers and, 265
short diagnostic mental
health interviews in, 59
Emotions. See Positive
emotion; Social-
emotional skills
Empathic engagement, and
therapeutic alliance, 6–7
Encopresis, **65,** 127–128, **183**
Engagement, in
psychotherapy, 268–269
Enuresis, 127, **183**
Escitalopram, 35, **288**
Etiology, and definition of
mental disorder, 64
Euphoria, and inhalant
intoxication, 156
Evidence-based principles, for
use of medications, 276
Excitement, and caffeine
intoxication, 147
Exclusion criteria, 84
Excoriation, 113
Exposure distress, and
posttraumatic stress
disorder, 114
Exposure therapy, for
anxiety, 40
Expressive language, and
development, 242
Extinction burst, 259

Facial features, and
neurobehavioral disorder
associated with prenatal
alcohol exposure, 28

Factitious disorder
intentionally produced
symptoms and, 189
recurrent and excessive
physical complaints
and, **42,** 43
somatic symptom disorder
and, 122
Family. See also Caregivers;
Parents
anxiety disorders and, 39
education about mental
health treatment for,
12–13
15-minute pediatric
diagnostic interview
and self-help
interventions for, 67–68
30-minute pediatric
diagnostic interview
and medical history
of, 78
Family therapy
description of and typical
indications for, **271**
irritable or labile mood
and, 37
Fantasy, and gender
dysphoria, 136
Fatigue
caffeine withdrawal and,
148
generalized anxiety
disorder and, 109
obstructive sleep apnea
and, 133
stimulant withdrawal and,
167
FDA. See Food and Drug
Administration
Fear
panic disorder and, 109

reactive attachment
disorder and, 117
specific phobia and, 106
of weight gain in anorexia
nervosa, 124
Fever, and opioid
withdrawal, 160
Fidgeting, and attention-
deficit/hyperactivity
disorder, 92
Fire setting, and conduct
disorder, 141
15-minute pediatric
diagnostic interview
diagnosis of probable or
unspecified disorders
and, 63–67
identification of leading
concerns in, 62–63
identifying and addressing
safety issues in, 63
prescreening of mental
health concerns and,
60–62
recommendation of next
step and, 67–69
Five-factor model, of
personality disorders, 222
Flashbacks, and
posttraumatic stress
disorder, 114
Flulike symptoms, and
caffeine withdrawal, 148
Fluoxetine, 35, 40, **287**
Fluvoxamine, **288**
Follow-up
DSM-5 pediatric
diagnostic interview
and, 83–84
15-minute pediatric
diagnostic interview
and, 69
psychotherapy and, 269

30-minute pediatric
diagnostic interview
and, 80
Food and Drug
Administration (FDA),
276, 277
Forgetfulness, and attention-
deficit/hyperactivity
disorder, 92
Fragile X syndrome, and
developmental delay, **26,**
28
Functional analysis of
behavior, 28–29, 259–260
Functional impairment, and
definition of mental
disorder, 64

Gait, inhalant intoxication
and unsteady, 156
Gambling disorder, 172–173
Gastrointestinal disturbance,
and caffeine intoxication,
148. *See also* Nausea
Gender dysphoria, 135–138
Genetic testing, and
developmental delays, 28
Generalized anxiety disorder
abbreviated DSM-5 criteria
for, **180**
anxious or avoidant
behavior and, **38,** 39
alternative diagnoses for,
110
DSM-5 pediatric
diagnostic interview
and, 109–110
medications for, **287–288**
prevalence of, **20**
shorthand description of, **65**
sleep problems and, **45**
Generalized Anxiety
Disorder 7-item scale, 56

Global developmental delay, 87
Global functioning, and rating scales, **229**
Goal-directed activity, and bipolar disorder, 98, 100
Grandiosity, and bipolar disorder, 97, 99
Group therapy, **271**
Guanfacine, 31, **286**
Guidelines. *See* Recommendations

Hallucinations
  alcohol withdrawal and, 147
  mental status examination and, 196
  schizophrenia and, 94
  sedative, hypnotic, or anxiolytic withdrawal and, 163
Hallucinogens. *See* Phencyclidine or other hallucinogen intoxication; Phencyclidine or other hallucinogen use disorder
Haloperidol, 277
Hand tremor, and sedative, hypnotic, or anxiolytic withdrawal, 163
Headache, and caffeine withdrawal, 148
Hearing. *See* Sensory impairment
Heat sensations, and panic disorder, 108
Herbal medicines, 191
Hierarchical ordering, of problem list, 252
Hoarding disorder, 112
Hospitalization

for psychosis or suicidality in parents, 57
  suicidality and, 48–49, 57
Humor, and therapeutic alliance, 7–8
Hydroxyzine, 46
Hyperactivity
  attention-deficit/ hyperactivity disorder and, 92
  sedative, hypnotic, or anxiolytic withdrawal and, 163
Hyperreactivity, and autism spectrum disorder, 90
Hypersomnia, and stimulant withdrawal, 167
Hypersomnolence disorder, 130–131
Hypervigilance, and posttraumatic stress disorder, 115
Hypocretin deficiency, and narcolepsy, 131
Hyporeactivity, and autism spectrum disorder, 90
Hypothyroidism, and withdrawn or sad mood, 32, **33**

ICD-10, and codes/coding, 85, 173, 234, 235, **236–240,** 252, **299**
Ideas of reference, and mental status examination, 197
Illness anxiety disorder, 122–123
Illusions, and mental status examination, 196–197
Immature defense mechanism, and developmental assessment, 190

Inattention. *See also* Attention
attention-deficit/
hyperactivity disorder
and, 92
Level 1 Cross-Cutting
Symptom Measure
and, **210**
Incoordination
inhalant intoxication and,
156
phencyclidine or other
hallucinogen
intoxication and, 154
Infants, diagnostic systems
for, 235. *See also*
Developmental history
Inhalant intoxication, 156–157
Inhalant use disorder, 154–156
Insight, and mental status
examination, 197
Insomnia, and insomnia
disorder
alcohol withdrawal and, 147
caffeine intoxication and,
147
medications for, 45, 46
opioid withdrawal and, 160
sedative, hypnotic, or
anxiolytic withdrawal
and, 163
sleep hygiene and, 43–44
stimulant withdrawal and,
167
symptoms of, 128–129
tobacco withdrawal and,
169
Integration, of mental and
physical health services,
303–304
Intellectual disability
abbreviated DSM-5 criteria
for, **176**

alternative diagnoses for,
87–88
developmental delay and,
26, 243
DSM-5 pediatric diagnostic
interview and, 86–88
modifiers for, 86
poor academic performance
and, 22, **23,** 24
Intentionally produced
symptoms, 189
Intermittent explosive
disorder, 139–140, **184**
International Classification of
Diseases. *See* ICD-10
Interpersonal relationships.
See also Social-emotional
skills; Social history
autism spectrum disorder
and, 89
substance-related and
addictive disorders
and, 144, 149, 152, 155,
157, 160–161, 164, 168,
170, 172
30-minute pediatric
diagnostic interview
and, 72–73
Interrupting, and attention-
deficit/hyperactivity
disorder, 93
IQ tests, 22, 24
Irritable mood, and irritability
caffeine withdrawal and,
148
cannabis withdrawal and,
151
as common clinical concern,
35–37
gambling disorder and, 172
generalized anxiety
disorder and, 110

Irritable mood, and
    irritability *(continued)*
    Level 1 Cross-Cutting
        Symptom Measure
        and, **210**
    major depressive disorder
        and, 104–105
    oppositional defiant
        disorder and, 138
    posttraumatic stress
        disorder and, 115
    reactive attachment
        disorder and, 117
    tobacco withdrawal and,
        169
Isotretinoin, 32

Judgment, and mental status
    examination, 197

Kleptomania, 143

Labile mood, as common
    clinical concern, 35–37
Lacrimation, and opioid
    withdrawal, 159
Language disorder, and
    intellectual disability, 87.
    See also Communication
    disorder; Speech
Lethargy, and inhalant
    intoxication, 156
Level 1 and Level 2 Cross-
    Cutting Symptom
    Measures, 60–61, 200–
    201, **202–211**
Level of Personality
    Functioning Scale, 222
Lies and lying. *See also*
    Factitious disorder;
    Malingering

conduct disorder and, 141
    gambling disorder and, 172
Life distractions, and poor
    academic performance,
    24
Lisdexamfetamine, **284**
Listening
    attention-deficit/
        hyperactivity disorder
        and, 92
    30-minute pediatric
        diagnostic interview
        and, 75
Lithium, 57

Major depressive disorder.
    See also Depression
    abbreviated DSM-5 criteria
        for, **179**
    alternative diagnoses for,
        103–104
    DSM-5 pediatric diagnostic
        interview and, 102–105
    eating disorders and, **55**
    irritable or labile mood
        and, **36**
    medications for, **287–288**
    modifiers for, 103
    postpartum maternal
        mental health and, **57**
    prevalence of, **20**
    self-harm or suicidality
        and, **47,** 49
    shorthand description of, **65**
    sleep problems and, **45**
    withdrawn or sad mood
        and, **33,** 35
Malingering. *See also*
    Factitious disorder

intentionally produced
symptoms and
differential diagnosis
of, 189
recurrent and excessive
physical complaints
and, 43
Marijuana, 51
Maternal peripartum
depression, 54–55, **231**
Medical conditions and
diseases. *See also* Medical
records; Physical
complaints; Primary care
physicians
anxiety disorder due to, 110
bipolar disorder due to, 99
depressive disorder due to,
104
differential diagnosis and
symptoms related to,
191–192
eating disorders and, **55**
obsessive-compulsive
disorder due to, 112
poor academic performance
and, 25
psychological factors
affecting, 122
30-minute pediatric
diagnostic interview
and, 78–79
withdrawn or sad mood
and, 32, **33**
Medical records, and adverse
effects of medications,
298, **299**

Medications. *See also*
Antipsychotics; Selective
serotonin reuptake
inhibitors; Self-
medication; Side effects;
Stimulants
appropriate prescription of
in community settings,
14–15
for attention-deficit/
hyperactivity
disorder, **278–286**
for depressive and anxiety
disorders, **287–289**
disruptive or aggressive
behavior and, 31
evidence-based principles
for prescription of, 276
15-minute pediatric
diagnostic interview
and, 68
frequency of use of
psychotropic, 275
irritable or labile mood
and, 37
key questions before
prescription of, 276–277
monitoring of for adverse
effects, 277, 293, 296–
298
for postpartum depression
or anxiety, 56, 57
psychotherapy combined
with, 268
recording of adverse
effects of, 298, **299**
self-harm or suicidality
and, 49
sleep problems and, 45–46
standard practices and,
275–276
Melatonin, 46, 68

Memory
mental status examination
and, 197
opioid intoxication and, 159
posttraumatic stress
disorder and, 114, 115
Mental health care. *See also*
Community behavioral
health systems; Early
intervention services;
Primary care physicians;
Treatment
barriers to for children, 9
integration of care and,
303–304
referrals for, 67
Mental status examination,
79, 195–197
Methylphenidate, 277, **278,
281, 282, 283**
Mini-mental state
examination, 79–80
Mirtazapine, 46
Misdiagnosis, and irritable or
labile mood, 35
Modified Checklist for
Autism in Toddlers (M-
CHAT), **231**
Modifiers. *See specific disorders*
Monitoring, of medications
for adverse effects, 277,
293, **294,** 296–298
Mood. *See also* Anger;
Irritable or labile mood;
Mood disorders;
Withdrawn or sad mood
caffeine withdrawal and
dysphoric or
depressed, 148
cannabis withdrawal and
depressed, 151

opioid withdrawal and
dysphoria, 159
review of systems in 30-
minute pediatric
diagnostic interview
and, 76–77
stimulant withdrawal and
dysphoric, 166
tobacco withdrawal and
depressed, 169
Mood disorders, and poor
academic performance,
23. *See also* Depression;
Mood
Motivation. *See also*
Motivational
interviewing
poor academic performance
and, 24
treatment for substance
abuse and, 54
Motivational interviewing, **273**
Motor skills. *See also* Muscles;
Psychomotor agitation;
Psychomotor retardation
developmental delays in,
27, **246–247**
identification of
developmental
milestones and, 241–
242, **244–245**
Multiaxial system, of
diagnosis in earlier
versions of DSM, 249–250
Multistep approach, to
diagnosis in community
settings, 12
Muscles. *See also* Motor skills
caffeine intoxication and
twitching of, 148

generalized anxiety disorder and tension in, 110

inhalant intoxication and weakness of, 156

opioid intoxication and aches in, 159

stimulant intoxication and weakness of, 166

Narcolepsy, 131–132

National Comorbidity Survey, 16, **20**

National Stressful Events Survey Acute Stress Disorder Short Scale, **232**

National Stressful Events Survey PTSD Short Scale, **232**

Nausea. *See also* Gastrointestinal disturbance

alcohol withdrawal and, 147

opioid withdrawal and, 159

panic disorder and, 108

sedative, hypnotic, or anxiolytic withdrawal and, 163

stimulant intoxication and, 166

Negative affect, and personality disorders, 222

Negative symptoms, of schizophrenia, 95

Neglect, childhood. *See also* Abuse

conflict with caregiver and, 191

Early Development and Home Background form and, 214

15-minute pediatric diagnostic interview and, 63

poor academic performance and, 24

Neologisms, and mental status examination, 196

Nervousness, and caffeine intoxication, 147

Neurobehavioral disorder associated with prenatal alcohol exposure, **26**, 28, 145–146

Neurodegenerative conditions, and developmental delay, **26**

Neurodevelopmental disorders

abbreviated DSM-5 criteria for, **176**

DSM-5 pediatric diagnostic interview and, 85–94

Neuroleptic malignant syndrome, 297

Nightmare disorder, 134. *See also* Dreams

Non–rapid eye movement sleep arousal disorders, 134

Nonverbal communicative behaviors, and autism spectrum disorder, 89

Not otherwise specified (NOS) condition, use of term, 64, 66

Nutritional deficiency, and avoidant/restrictive food intake disorder, 125

Nystagmus, and inhalant intoxication, 156

Obsessions
mental status examination
and, 196
obsessive-compulsive
disorder and, 111
30-minute pediatric
diagnostic interview
and, 77
Obsessive-compulsive
disorder (OCD)
abbreviated DSM-5 criteria
for, **180**
alternative diagnoses for,
112
anxious or avoidant
behavior and, **38,** 40
DSM-5 pediatric
diagnostic interview
and, 110–113
medications for, **287–289**
modifiers for, 111–112
shorthand description of, **66**
Obstructive sleep apnea, 44–
45, 132–133
OCD. *See* Obsessive-
compulsive disorder
ODD. *See* Oppositional
defiant disorder
Olanzapine, **282**
Opioid intoxication, 159
Opioid use disorder, 157–159
Opioid withdrawal, 159–160
Oppositional defiant
disorder (ODD)
abbreviated DSM-5 criteria
for, **184**
behavior management
training for, 31, 268, **272**
cognitive-behavioral
therapy for, **270**
conduct disorder and, 142

disruptive or aggressive
behavior and, 29, **30,** 31
DSM-5 pediatric
diagnostic interview
and, 138–139
irritable or labile mood
and, **36**
poor academic
performance and, **23**
shorthand description of, **66**
social skills training for, **273**
Other specified disorder, use
of term, 66–67
Other (or unknown) substance
intoxication, 171–172
Other (or unknown) substance
use disorder, 169–171
Other (or unknown) substance
withdrawal, 171–172
Over-the-counter
medications, 191

Paliperidone, **282**
Palpitations, and panic
disorder, 108
Panic attacks
isolated as short-term
anxiety symptom, 39
recurrent and excessive
physical complaints
and, **42**
shorthand description of, **66**
as specifier for panic
disorder, 109
Panic disorder
abbreviated DSM-5 criteria
for, **179**
alternative diagnoses for,
109
anxious or avoidant
behavior and, **38,** 39

DSM-5 pediatric
diagnostic interview
and, 108–109
prevalence of, **20**
Parents. *See also* Caregivers;
Family
anxious or avoidant
behavior and, 39, 40
influence of mental health
on children, 56
successful use of special
time by, 258–259
therapeutic alliance and, 6, 8
Parent training. *See* Behavior
management training
Paresthesias, and panic
disorder, 108
Paroxetine, **288**
Patient Health Questionnaire-
9, 56, **230, 232**
Patients
self-help strategies for in
community settings, 13
treatment plans and goals
of, 253–255
Pediatric approvals, by FDA,
276
Pediatric Symptom Checklist
(PSC), 60, **229**
Persistent depressive
disorder (dysthymia)
major depressive disorder
and, 103
self-harm or suicidality
and, **47**
withdrawn or sad mood
and, 32, **33**
Personality disorders. *See also*
Personality Inventory
for DSM-5—Brief
Form—Child Age 11–17

dimensional model of,
222–223
immature defense
mechanism and, 190
Personality Inventory for
DSM-5—Brief Form—
Child Age 11–17, 221–
223, **224–226**
Personality Trait Rating
Form, 222
Phencyclidine or other
hallucinogen
intoxication, 153–154
Phencyclidine or other
hallucinogen use
disorder, 152–153
Phobias. *See also* Specific
phobia
mental status examination
and, 196
shorthand description of, **66**
Physical complaints. *See also*
Medical conditions;
Somatic complaints
anxious or avoidant
behavior and, 39
recurrent and excessive as
common clinical
concern, 40–43
Physiological reactions, and
posttraumatic stress
disorder, 114
Pica, 126, **183**
Picture exchange system, 28
Play
gender dysphoria and, 136
special time and child-
directed, 258
*Pocket Guide to the DSM-5
Diagnostic Exam, The*
(Nussbaum 2013), 3, 4

Positive emotion
    posttraumatic stress
        disorder and, 115
    reactive attachment
        disorder and, 117
Postcrisis planning, for
    caregivers, 263–265
Postpartum depression. *See*
    Maternal peripartum
    depression
Posttraumatic stress disorder
    (PTSD)
    abbreviated DSM-5 criteria
        for, **181–182**
    alternative diagnoses for,
        116–117
    anxious or avoidant
        behavior and, **38,** 40
    blame and, 115
    cognitive-behavioral
        therapy for, **270**
    disruptive or aggressive
        behavior and, 29, **30**
    DSM-5 pediatric
        diagnostic interview
        and, 114–117
    irritable or labile mood
        and, 35, **36**
    modifiers for, 115
    prevalence of, **20**
    rating scales for, **230**
    shorthand description of, **66**
    sleep problems and, **45**
Practice guidelines, and
    treatment goals, 255. *See
    also* Recommendations
Pregnancy, medication
    choices during, 57
Pre-interview assessment
    tools, 60–62
Premenstrual dysphoric
    disorder, 104

Prenatal alcohol exposure. *See*
    Neurobehavioral
    disorder associated with
    prenatal alcohol exposure
Preoccupation
    gambling disorder and, 172
    illness anxiety disorder
        and, 123
Preschool children, and age-
    based behavioral
    screening, 17, **18–19**
Prevalence. *See also specific
    disorders*
    of mental disorders in
        adolescents, **20**
    of self-harm and suicidality
        in adolescents, 46
    of substance abuse in
        adolescents, 49
Primary care physicians
    appropriate prescription of
        medications in
        community settings
        by, 14–15
    limited mental health
        training of, 21, 200
    recommendations for
        approach of to child
        mental health
        treatment, 15
    short diagnostic mental
        health interviews by, 59
Problem lists, and diagnosis,
    249–252
Provisional diagnosis, 252
Psychiatric history, and 30-
    minute pediatric
    diagnostic interview, 75–
    76
Psychological factors
    affecting other medical
    conditions, 122

Psychomotor agitation. *See also* Restlessness
    alcohol withdrawal and, 147
    caffeine intoxication and, 148
    sedative, hypnotic, or anxiolytic withdrawal and, 163
    stimulant intoxication and, 166
    stimulant withdrawal and, 167
Psychomotor retardation
    inhalant intoxication and, 156
    stimulant intoxication and, 166
    stimulant withdrawal and, 167
Psychopharmacology. *See* Medications
Psychosis. *See also* Psychoticism; Schizophrenia spectrum and other psychotic disorders
    Level 1 Cross-Cutting Symptom Measure and, **211**
    postpartum maternal mental health and, **57**
    30-minute pediatric diagnostic interview and, 77
Psychosocial functioning. *See also* Social-emotional skills
    avoidant/restrictive food intake disorder and, 125
    rating scales for difficulties in, **229**
Psychosocial interventions
    behavioral activation as, 260–261
    bullying and, 261–262
    functional analysis of behavior and, 259–260
    postcrisis planning for caregivers and, 263–265
    sleep hygiene and, 262–263
    special time as, 258–259
    time-outs as, 257–258
Psychotherapy. *See also* Cognitive-behavioral therapy
    anxiety and, 40
    choice of techniques for, 267–269
    depression and, 34
    commonly recommended methods of, **270–273**
    initiation of in community settings, 14
    postpartum depression or anxiety and, 56
    self-harm or suicidality and, 49
Psychotic disorder(s), 96, **290–292.** *See also* Schizophrenia spectrum and other psychotic disorders
Psychoticism, and personality disorders, 222
PTSD. *See* Posttraumatic stress disorder
Pupillary dilation
    opioid withdrawal and, 160
    phencyclidine or other hallucinogen intoxication and, 154
    stimulant intoxication and, 166
Pyromania, 142–143

Quetiapine, 46, **291**

Rapid eye movement sleep behavior disorder, 135
Rapid eye movement (REM) sleep latency, and narcolepsy, 131
Rating scales. *See also* Structured interviews
developmental milestones and, 22
importance of understanding limitations of, 62
list of validated and free for use with children and adolescents, **229–231**
pre-interview assessment tools and, 60–62
principles for use of, 227–228
screening process in community settings and, 11
for severity of specific disorders, **232–233**
RDoC. *See* Research Domain Criteria
Reactive attachment disorder, 117–118, **180**
Receptive language, and development, 242
Recklessness, and posttraumatic stress disorder, 115
Recommendations
for clinical practice, 301–302
for education, 302–303
for initiating therapeutic alliance with child, 8

for next step in treatment after 15-minute pediatric diagnostic interview, 67–69
for primary care approach to child mental health treatment, 15
for research, 303
for use of rating scales, 227–228
Relaxation training, **273**
Repetitive thoughts and behaviors
DSM-5 pediatric diagnostic interview and, 84
Level 1 Cross-Cutting Symptom Measure and, **211**
Research, recommendations on, 303
Research Diagnostic Criteria–Preschool Age (RDC-PA), 235
Research Domain Criteria (RdoC), 234–235
Restless legs syndrome, 133–135
Restlessness. *See also* Fidgeting; Psychomotor agitation
caffeine intoxication and, 147
cannabis withdrawal and, 151
generalized anxiety disorder and, 109
tobacco withdrawal and, 169
Restricted interests, and autism spectrum disorder, 90

Rhinorrhea, and opioid
   withdrawal, 159
Risk factors, for suicidality, 48
Risky behaviors
   bipolar disorder and, 98, 100
   substance-related and
      addictive disorders
      and, 144, 149, 152, 155,
      157, 161, 164, 168, 170
Risperidone, 31, 46, **290**, 296
Ruminant disorder, 126
Running away, and conduct
   disorder, 141

Sadness, and reactive
   attachment disorder, 117.
   See also Withdrawn or
   sad mood
Safety. *See also* Self-harm;
   Suicide and suicidality
   disruptive or aggressive
      behavior and, **30**
   15-minute pediatric
      diagnostic interview
      and, 63, 68
   postpartum maternal
      mental health and, **57**
   substance abuse and, **50**
   30-minute pediatric
      diagnostic interview
      and, 76
   withdrawn or sad mood
      and, 34
Schizoaffective disorder, 96,
   177
Schizophrenia
   abbreviated DSM-5 criteria
      for, **177**
   alternative diagnoses for,
      95–97
   DSM-5 pediatric diagnostic
      interview and, 94–97

modifiers for, 95
Schizophrenia spectrum and
   other psychotic disorders.
   See also Psychotic
   disorders; Schizophrenia
   abbreviated DSM-5 criteria
      for, **177**
   DSM-5 pediatric diagnostic
      interview and, 94–97
   medications for, **290–292**
Schizophreniform disorder, 96
School(s). *See also* Education
   conduct disorder and
      truancy from, 141
   15-minute pediatric
      diagnostic interview
      and recommendations
      for assessment in, 68
   poor academic performance
      as common clinical
      concern and, 22–25
School-age children, and age-
   based behavioral
   screening, 17, **18–19**
Screen for Child Anxiety
   Related Emotional
   Disorders (SCARED), **229**
Screening, and screening
   questions
   age-based for behavioral
      health in community
      settings, 17
   anxious or avoidant
      behavior and, **38**
   bipolar and related
      disorders and, 97
   depressive disorders and,
      101–102, 104–105
   developmental delay and,
      26
   disruptive or aggressive
      behavior and, **30**

Screening, and screening
   questions (*continued*)
   disruptive, impulse-
      control, and conduct
      disorders and, 137–138
   eating disorders and, **55,** 123
   elimination disorders and,
      126–127
   gender dysphoria and,
      135–136
   irritable or labile mood
      and, **36**
   Level 1 and 2 Cross-
      Cutting Symptom
      Measures and, 200
   for maternal depressive and
      anxiety problems, 56
   for mental distress in
      community settings,
      10–11
   neurodevelopmental
      disorders and, 86
   obsessive-compulsive
      disorder and, 110–111
   poor academic
      performance and, **23**
   postpartum maternal
      mental health and, **57**
   preassessment tools for,
      60–62
   recurrent and excessive
      physical complaints
      and, **42**
   schizophrenia spectrum
      and other psychotic
      disorders and, 94
   self-harm or suicidality
      and, **47**
   sleep problems and, **45,** 128
   somatic symptom and
      related disorders and,
      120–121

   substance-related and
      addictive disorders
      and, **50,** 143–144
   trauma- and stressor-related
      disorders and, 113–114
   withdrawn or sad mood
      and, **33**
Sedative drugs, 51
Sedative, hypnotic, or
   anxiolytic intoxication,
   162–163
Sedative, hypnotic, or
   anxiolytic use disorder,
   160–162
Sedative, hypnotic, or
   anxiolytic withdrawal,
   163
Seizures
   alcohol withdrawal and, 147
   sedative, hypnotic, or
      anxiolytic withdrawal
      and, 163
   stimulant intoxication
      and, 166
Selective mutism, 107
Selective serotonin reuptake
   inhibitors (SSRIs)
   anxious or avoidant
      behavior and, 40
   monitoring of, **296**
   postpartum depression or
      anxiety and, 56, 57
   self-harm or suicidality
      and, 49
   side effects of, 293, **295,** 296
   withdrawn or sad mood
      and, 34–35
Self-esteem, and bipolar
   disorder, 97, 99. *See also*
   Self-image
Self-harm. *See also* Safety;
   Suicide and suicidality

anxious or avoidant
behavior and, **38**
as common clinical
concern, 46–49
dialectical behavior
therapy for, **271**
eating disorders and, **55**
15-minute pediatric
diagnostic interview
and, 63
postcrisis planning for
caregivers and, 264
withdrawn or sad mood
and, 32, **33**
Self-help strategies
15-minute pediatric
diagnostic interview
and, 67–68
teaching of to patients and
caregivers, 13
Self-image, and posttraumatic
stress disorder, 115. *See
also* Self-esteem
Self-medication, and
substance abuse, **50**
Sensory impairment. *See also*
Vision
developmental delay and,
26, 27
poor academic
performance and, **23**
Separation anxiety disorder
abbreviated DSM-5 criteria
for, **179**
anxious or avoidant
behavior and, **38**, 39
prevalence of, **20**
Serotonin syndrome, 293
Sertraline, 35, 40, **287**
Severity, and rating scales for
specific disorders, 228,
232–233

Short Mood and Feelings
Questionnaire (SMFQ),
230
Side effects, of medications
ICD-10-CM codes for, **299**
monitoring of, 277, 293,
296–298
recording of, 298
Sleep problems. *See also*
Sleep-wake disorders
bipolar disorder and, 97, 99
cannabis withdrawal and,
151
as common clinical
concern, 43–46
generalized anxiety
disorder and, 110
Level 1 Cross-Cutting
Symptom Measure
and, **210**
posttraumatic stress
disorder and, 116
sleep hygiene and
psychosocial
interventions for, 262–
263
30-minute pediatric
diagnostic interview
and, 78
Sleep-related hypoventilation,
and obstructive sleep
apnea, 133
Sleep-wake disorders, 128–
135. *See also* Sleep
problems
SNAP-IV-C Rating Scale, **230**
Social anxiety disorder
disruptive behavior and, 29
specific phobia and, 108

Social-emotional skills. *See also*
Interpersonal
relationships;
Psychosocial functioning;
Psychosocial
interventions; Social
history; Social skills
training
autism spectrum disorder
and, 89
development of, 27, 242,
244–247
rating scales and, **229**
reactive attachment
disorder and, 117
Social history. *See also*
Interpersonal
relationships; Social-
emotional skills
symptoms related to
developmental conflict
or stage and, 190
30-minute pediatric
diagnostic interview
and, 78–79
Social (pragmatic)
communication
disorder, 88
Social skills training, **273**. *See
also* Social-emotional
skills
Somatic complaints. *See also*
Physical complaints
cannabis withdrawal and,
151
Level 1 Cross-Cutting
Symptom Measure
and, **210**
30-minute pediatric
diagnostic interview
and, 78
Somatic symptom disorder

alternative diagnoses for,
121–122
DSM-5 pediatric diagnostic
interview and, 121–122
modifiers for, 121
recurrent and excessive
physical complaints
and, **42**
Somatic symptom and related
disorders
DSM-5 pediatric diagnostic
interview and, 120–123
intentionally produced
symptoms and, 189
treatments for, 41, 43
Special education program, 24
Special time, as psychosocial
intervention, 258–259
Specificity, of diagnosis, 251–
252
Specific learning disorder
abbreviated DSM-5 criteria
for, **177**
intellectual disability and,
88
poor academic performance
and, **23,** 24
Specific phobia
alternative diagnoses for,
107–108
anxious or avoidant
behavior and, **38,** 39
DSM-5 pediatric diagnostic
interview and, 106–108
modifiers for, 107
shorthand description of, **66**
Specifiers. *See specific disorders*
Speech. *See also*
Communication
disorder; Language
disorder

attention-deficit/
hyperactivity disorder
and, 92
bipolar disorder and, 97, 100
developmental milestones
and, 242, **244–245**
inhalant intoxication and
slurred, 156
mental status examination
and, 196
opioid intoxication and
slurred, 159
schizophrenia and
disorganized, 95
Speech sound disorder, 87
Spence Children's Anxiety
Scale (SCAS), **229**
Spence Preschool Anxiety
Scale, **229**
Startle, posttraumatic stress
disorder and
exaggerated, 115
Stepwise approach, to
differential diagnosis,
189–193
Stereotyped or repetitive
speech, and autism
spectrum disorder, 89
Stereotypic movement
disorder, 90–91
Stimulant(s)
monitoring of, **294**
side effects of, 293, **294**
substance abuse and, 51
Stimulant intoxication, 165–
166
Stimulant use disorder, 163–
165
Stimulant withdrawal, 166–
167

Strengths and Difficulties
Questionnaire (SDQ),
60, **229**
Structured interviews,
disadvantages of, 73
Stupor, and inhalant
intoxication, 156
Substance Abuse and Mental
Health Services
Administration, 268
Substance/medication-
induced anxiety
disorder, 110
Substance/medication-
induced bipolar
disorder, 99
Substance/medication-
induced depressive
disorder, 104
Substance/medication-
induced obsessive-
compulsive disorder, 112
Substance/medication-
induced psychotic
disorder, 96
Substance/medication-
induced sleep disorders,
130, 131, 135
Substance abuse. *See also*
Substance-related and
addictive disorders;
Substance use disorder
as common clinical
concern, 49–54
differential diagnosis and
symptoms related to,
191
irritable or labile mood
and, **36**
Level 1 Cross-Cutting
Symptom Measure
and, **211**

Substance abuse *(continued)*
  rating scales for, **230**
  30-minute pediatric
    diagnostic interview
    and, 78
  withdrawn or sad mood
    and, 32, **33**, 34
Substance-related and
    addictive disorders,
    143–173. *See also*
    Substance abuse;
    Substance use disorder
Substance use disorder. *See
    also* Substance abuse;
    Substance-related and
    addictive disorders
  alternative diagnoses for,
    145–146, 148, 150, 153,
    156, 158–159, 162, 165,
    169
  cognitive-behavioral
    therapy for, **270**
  eating disorders and, **55**
  family therapy for, **271**
  modifiers for, 145, 147, 150,
    151, 153, 155–156, 158,
    159, 161–162, 163, 165,
    166, 167, 168, 171
  motivational interviewing
    for, **273**
  poor academic performance
    and, **23**
  screening for, **50**
  self-harm or suicidality
    and, **47**
Substance withdrawal,
    screening questions for,
    50
Suicide and suicidality. *See
    also* Safety
  as common clinical
    concern, 46–49

dialectical behavior
    therapy for, **271**
  15-minute pediatric
    diagnostic interview
    and, 63, 68
  irritable or labile mood and,
    36
  Level 1 Cross-Cutting
    Symptom Measure
    and, **211**
  postpartum maternal
    mental health and, **57**
  withdrawn or sad mood
    and, 32, 34
Supplemental questions, and
    Cultural Formulation
    Interview, 213–214
Sweating
  panic disorder and, 108
  phencyclidine or other
    hallucinogen
    intoxication and, 154
  stimulant intoxication
    and, 166
Symptoms. *See also* Exclusion
    criteria; *specific disorders*
  caregiver conflict and, 190–
    191
  comorbidity of mental
    disorders and, 192–193
  developmental conflict or
    stage and, 190
  intentional production of,
    189
  medical conditions and,
    191–192

Tachycardia
  caffeine intoxication and,
    148
  cannabis intoxication and,
    151

phencyclidine or other hallucinogen intoxication and, 154

stimulant intoxication and, 166

Tantrums
disruptive behavior and, 29
functional analysis of behavior and, 259

Tardive dyskinesia, 297–298

TF-CBT. *See* Trauma-focused cognitive-behavioral therapy

Theft, and conduct disorder, 140, 141

Therapeutic alliance
Cultural Formulation Interview and, 201
as first step in successful diagnosis and treatment, 5–8
intentionally produced symptoms and, 189
neurobehavioral disorder associated with prenatal alcohol exposure and, 28
psychotherapy and, 269
30-minute pediatric diagnostic interview and, 71–74

Thioridazine, 277

30-minute pediatric diagnostic interview
confidentiality and, 74–75
follow-up questions and, 80
listening and, 75
medical history and, 78–79
mental status examination and, 79
mini-mental state examination and, 79–80

presentation of current illness and, 75
psychiatric history and, 75–76
review of systems and, 76–78
safety issues and, 76
therapeutic alliance and, 71–74

Thought, and thinking
bipolar disorder and, 98, 100
mental status examination and, 196
obsessive-compulsive disorder and, 111
somatic symptom disorder and, 121

Tic disorders, 91, 293

Time
other (or unknown) substance use disorder and, 170
short diagnostic interviews and constraints on, 59–60
somatic symptom disorder and excessive investment in health concerns, 121

Time-outs, and psychosocial interventions, 257–258

Tobacco use disorder, 167–169

Tobacco withdrawal, 169

Toddlers, diagnostic systems for, 235

Tolerance
cannabis use disorder and, 149–150
opioid use disorder and, 158
other (or unknown) substance use disorder and, 170

Tolerance *(continued)*
  phencyclidine or other
      hallucinogen use
      disorder and, 152–153
  sedative, hypnotic, or
      anxiolytic use disorder
      and, 161
  stimulant use disorder
      and, 164
  tobacco use disorder and,
      168
Tourette's disorder, 91
Transient regression, 190
Trauma. *See also* Trauma- and
      stressor-related disorders
  anxious or avoidant
      behavior and, **38**
  30-minute pediatric
      diagnostic interview
      and, 77
Trauma-focused cognitive-
      behavioral therapy (TF-
      CBT), 268, **270**
Trauma- and stressor-related
      disorders. *See also* Trauma
  abbreviated DSM-5 criteria
      for, **180–182**
  DSM-5 pediatric diagnostic
      interview and, 113–118
Treatment. *See also*
      Community behavioral
      health systems; Follow-
      up; Hospitalization;
      Medications;
      Psychosocial
      interventions;
      Psychotherapy;
      Screening; Treatment
      plans; *specific disorders*

  15-minute pediatric
      diagnostic interview
      and recommendations
      for, 67–69
  integration of care and,
      303–304
  Level 2 Cross-Cutting
      Symptom Measure
      and assessment of
      progress in, 201
  of parental mental health
      problems during
      child's early
      development phase, 56
  therapeutic alliance as first
      step in successful, 6–8
  underuse of during
      childhood, 9
Treatment plans
  development of, 2 49, **256**
  initiation of in community
      settings, 13
  patient or caregiver goals
      and, 253–255
Trembling, and panic disorder,
      108
Tremor
  inhalant intoxication and,
      156
  phencyclidine or other
      hallucinogen
      intoxication and, 154
Trichotillomania, 113
Tricyclic antidepressants, 276

Unspecified disorder, use of
      term, 66–67
Urine drug testing, and
      substance abuse, 51

Validity, of rating scales, 228
Valproate, 57
Vanderbilt ADHD Diagnostic
    Parent Rating Scale/
    Vanderbilt ADHD
    Diagnostic Teacher
    Rating Scale, **230**
Vindictiveness, and
    oppositional defiant
    disorder, 139
Violence
  conduct disorder and, 140
  intermittent explosive
    disorder and, 139
Vision. *See also* Pupillary
    dilation; Sensory
    impairment
  inhalant intoxication and
    blurring of, 156
  phencyclidine or other
    hallucinogen
    intoxication and
    blurring of, 154
Visual motor problem
    solving, 242, **244–245**

Weight gain or loss
  anorexia nervosa and fear
    of, 124

avoidant/restrictive food
    intake disorder and, 125
  as side effect of
    antipsychotics, 296
  stimulant intoxication
    and, 166
Withdrawal, and substance-
    related and addictive
    disorders, 145, 150, 158,
    164–165, 168, 170–171
Withdrawn or sad mood, as
    common clinical
    concern, 32–35
Work environment, and poor
    academic performance,
    24
World Health Organization,
    234
Worry, and panic disorder,
    109

Yawning, and opioid
    withdrawal, 160

Z codes, and ICD-10, 235,
    236–240, 252
Zero to Three program, 68
Ziprasidone, **291**